— YOUR —

HEALTH

IS NON-NEGOTIABLE

YOUR SIX WEEK GUIDE
— TO —
TOTAL TRANSFORMATION

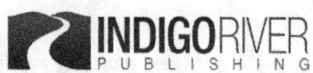

YOUR

HEALTH

IS NON-NEGOTIABLE

YOUR SIX WEEK GUIDE
— TO —
TOTAL TRANSFORMATION

SHERRY THACKER

Indigo River Publishing

Your Health Is Nonnegotiable: Your Six-Week Guide to Total Transformation

Copyright © 2018 by Sherry Thacker

Indigo River Publishing
3 West Garden Street, Ste. 352
Pensacola, FL 32502
www.indigoriverpublishing.com

Editors: Qat Wanders and Regina Cornell
Cover Design: 99 Designs
Interior Design: mycustombookcover.com
Creative Contributor: Christopher Morris

Ordering Information:

Quantity sales: Special discounts are available on quantity purchases by corporations, associations, and others. For details, contact the publisher at the address above. Orders by US trade bookstores and wholesalers: Please contact the publisher at the address above.

Printed in the United States of America

Library of Congress Control Number: 2018965688
ISBN: 978-1-948080-62-0

First Edition

With Indigo River Publishing, you can always expect great books, strong voices, and meaningful messages. Most importantly, you'll always find . . . words worth reading.

DEDICATION

To my super humans, Sylvie, Mara, and Eloise: You stood by me when I really needed you most, and you had my back for the whole ride! Your trust and belief in me empowered me when I was at my lowest. Together we have changed the lives of so many grateful people, including our own. I love you guys! xoxo

And of course to Jeff, my guardian angel: Words cannot express the amount of gratitude I have for the love and support that you give to me and our precious Liam every day. Not a day goes by where you don't watch over us, and we are truly blessed to have you in our lives.

Contents

Introduction 1

My Story 23

Fasting 33

Inflammation 67

Gut Health 95

Stress 115

Sleep 145

Detox and Cleanse 167

Conclusion 201

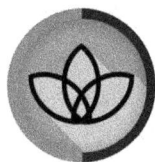

INTRODUCTION

Congratulations on taking action! Together we will embark on an amazing new journey. This book is not a diet plan or fitness program, and it doesn't promote any of the trendy temporary diets. (Yeah, they work for a little while, but then all the weight piles back on.) This is a six-week transformation because it promises to heal your body from the inside out.

Our message will particularly resonate with women who have lost themselves while caring for other people. We care for our children, husbands, parents, homes, and, of course, our colleagues and bosses. We spend every waking moment making sure everyone else is taken care of until that one day comes when we look in the mirror and don't recognize ourselves anymore.

We've lost our energy, drive, motivation, and our figures somewhere in the process of LIFE.

This book caters to all women who are tired of yo-yo dieting,

2 • YOUR HEALTH IS NON-NEGOTIABLE

tired of trying everything only to put all the weight back on. Women who are tired of all the mixed messages online. Tired of the overload of information and everyone telling you to take the complete opposite approach from the suggestions of the last person you spoke to. This book puts all the confusion to rest—for good.

This is an action-based book that will help you weed through all the noise that you are exposed to on the internet and television. You will learn the science of *your* body, and you will learn how to fuel and move your body the way it was originally designed. You will design your own lifestyle plan based on your genetics, environmental upbringing, stress levels, hormones, and everything that is YOU.

YOU University!

You're reading this guide because you are tired of health protocols that don't work and following the trendy diet of the month that you found on Pinterest or YouTube. You're probably tired of counting calories and points, and you're ready to invest some time and energy into transforming your mind, body, and spirit; the net result being a lifestyle transformation. Weight loss will be a mere side effect of everything that you learn during your transformation. So let's roll up our sleeves together. We have plenty of ground to cover.

Over the next six weeks, I will not *tell* you what to do. You are in total control of what you do with the information that is shared here. This guide is an actionable, educational tool that will help you to understand how your body works. It's just like reading your body's owner's manual! From there, we will help you understand what makes your body different from everyone else's. Your body *is* different. Your genetics, the environment you were raised in, the chemicals you have been exposed to your entire life, your hormones, your stress levels, your metabolism, your lifestyle, your age, your sleeping habits, your work—gasp! I could go on and on. All of this will impact how your body functions.

Science reveals that our microbiomes are, in fact, unique fingerprints of how our bodies function. The collection of bacteria is uniquely yours and very different from anyone else's. Since the moment our bodies left the womb, bacteria has infiltrated our bodies and established the makeup of our microbiomes. Because we all lead a unique lifestyle and so many factors can influence the dance and mixture of microbiota that live and die within us, scientists are only just starting to understand this fascinating world.

So, please understand, there's nothing "wrong" with you. So many women I speak to compare themselves to other women. They are envious of other women's genetics or their metabolisms or how "easy" some people have it when it comes to health. Be patient with your body and take time to study your body, understand it, test it, and then follow through to create your own set of instructions required to heal yourself after you have identified inflammatory foods that are causing inflammation in your body. You can do this by understanding the current condition of your gut health, your stress levels, sleeping patterns, and fitness activities.

Make an effort to learn about toxins in your home and in your working environment. I know it feels overwhelming now, but trust me, we will explore each of the factors in your body and lifestyle that could be preventing you from losing weight or causing you to be sick, and step by step, we will study them and correct them so you will essentially heal your body and create a new lifestyle for yourself that will support a healthy, pain-free future.

So over the next 42 days, be open-minded about experimenting with your body. Let your body do the talking. Your body will speak loud and clear on what it likes and what it doesn't like. Perhaps, up until now, you have just not been paying close attention to all the signals that your body sends you when it's not healthy and happy. Hopefully, we can change that.

Now, take a deep breath and release your fears. You may be a little nervous, and that's perfectly okay. We are chemically wired to resist change, stay in our comfort zone, and protect ourselves from change and danger. You have adopted a certain eating pattern and lifestyle throughout your entire life, and I venture to guess that, other than occasionally, you have not deviated from them very much.

Don't worry about making sudden changes—transformation won't happen overnight, and you make all the rules. This is your body, your science experiment, your test. Explore. Try to come to everything with an open mind. Learn as much as you can, and implement whatever fits most with your lifestyle and start from there.

At www.myhealthisnonnegotiable.com you will find extra videos and resources to help you on this journey. You can also join our free Facebook group to connect with our community: www.facebook.com/groups/sherrythackerfans/.

Let me take a moment to explain what kind of program my team and I have created online that has been transforming the lives of thousands of women. We have designed a program that helps women understand that it's time to make their health nonnegotiable after they have neglected their bodies while caring for other people. These women have woken up and acknowledged that their bodies are broken. We help heal the body from a cellular level using functional medicine strategies, live interactive online fitness classes, and weekly educational live mastermind meetings with yours truly.

The story-sharing and motivation of our thriving community helps our members stay accountable for setting their goals, creating a plan of implementation, and, of course, following through on said plan. In order to guarantee success, we assign each and every member their own private accountability coach who is there for her every step of the way, holding her hand and answering all the questions that she may have about the program. We also pair our members with someone who is also experiencing the program for the first time, in addition to someone who has graduated from the program to act as a mentor.

Because this program is designed 100 percent for your body's genetics, stress levels, and sleeping patterns, and you are designing your own lifestyle plan while experimenting with the science and strategies that we share with you, you absolutely cannot fail on this plan. Results are 100 percent guaranteed! To find out more information about this program, please visit my website at www.myhealthisnonnegotiable.com.

Your Why

Based on our online Six-Week Transformation Program, I can tell you that the people who have achieved the greatest results make their "whys" the biggest priority as they embark on this journey. Your why *must* be stronger than your need to taste that bagel with cream cheese, and your why can't just be about losing weight. For some reason, we all lose that battle between our belt and the bagel when the hunger hormone ghrelin takes over. (Yes, I know you may not be familiar with ghrelin yet, but we'll be going over that very shortly!)

Knowing your why helps you to create a set of standards. Once you understand the science, the knowledge suddenly becomes important to you because it becomes tangible. Resisting some types of food to avoid getting fat is one thing. Understanding how vegetable oil destroys your brain, how wheat and other chemicals disrupt your hormones, and so on, suddenly brings on a whole new meaning. Keeping your body clean ultimately becomes something that you believe in, helping to create a foundation for you to build upon.

Building a foundation, having something that you truly *believe* in, is the only true cure for that lack of discipline. Is it a lack of discipline? Maybe you've had an addiction to sugar for most of your life without really knowing it. The sugar addiction creates the unbearable cravings, the hormone imbalances, the weight gain, the brain fog, the joint pain . . . ummm, I'd better stop there for now, but I could go on.

Most of the people I meet are in a place in their lives where they just don't feel well anymore. They are tired, unmotivated, uninspired, overweight, and uncomfortable in their clothes and in their own skin. They have back, neck, shoulder, knee, and joint pain. Their whys could include:

- Pain relief

- Renewed energy

- Disease prevention

- Living a better life

- Improved cognitive performance

- Enhanced drive and motivation

What's your why?

The Goals of Our Program:

- Avoid sugars

- Avoid vegetable oils

- Create regimented feeding and fasting windows

- Identify inflammatory foods

- Heal the gut

- Manage stress

- Master a proper sleeping ritual

- Learn how to listen to the body

- Understand how the body works

- Create your own lifestyle (meal and fitness plan, stress and sleep management systems) that you will stick to no matter what life challenges come your way.

Preparing for the Six-Week Transformation Program

There are several aspects to this six-week transformation, so before we go any further, I'd just like to go over what you will experience and how it will benefit you.

Find a Buddy/Accountability Coach

As mentioned in the introduction, when you come into our community you are immediately paired up with an accountability coach, a spark buddy, someone who is new to our program and is ready to ignite! They are ready to make their health nonnegotiable, and they are excited to learn everything they can about the body. You are also paired with a flame buddy, someone who has graduated our program, wishes to continue to keep his or her health nonnegotiable, and has decided to become a guiding light for others joining our program, to help support you in your journey. We highly recommend that you find somebody who is like-minded and willing to walk through this journey with you in order to share your experience! You will likely have ups and downs—like everyone else—as life throws you challenges, and it's helpful to have someone who has gone through this program, or who is going through the same things, to help support you.

Choose Your Workouts

In our online course, you will discover virtual interactive workouts where my instructors can see you and you can see them. There is a wide variety of classes to choose from and times posted on our schedule. Moms find the virtual interactive workouts to be most beneficial, as they don't have to find someone to watch their kids when they need to take some time to go for a workout. We also have a wide variety of prerecorded workouts if you cannot attend the live ones. Regardless of whether you use our workout resources, make sure that you plan your workouts well in advance of what is marked on the calendar and make them nonnegotiable. Our online virtual workouts have been known to keep our clients extremely accountable, so we do recommend taking advantage of them. Go check out our program at www.myhealthisnonnegotiable.com.

Choose Your Recipes

You may have decided to pick up *Your Health Is Nonnegotiable Cookbook*, which accompanies this book and completely lays out the six-week process for you. In this book, each chapter reflects a corresponding week of the challenge. So as we cover fasting, we have suggested recipes to help you in your fast and to help you reach a state of ketosis. (Please consult your medical professional if you are diabetic or taking medications.) In week two, we suggest recipes to help you reduce inflammation in your body, and in week three we suggest fermented foods, live cultures, bone broth, and other beneficial foods that help you heal your gut. The cookbook will also give suggestions for juicing and detoxing in week six.

Go through Your Cupboards to Discover the Misleading Labels

It's time to dive into your fridge and cupboards! Let's make a deal, okay? You don't have to change anything *or* throw anything out—just yet. All that I ask that you do is to go through your inventory of food and lay everything out on the counter. Below you will find a list of the ingredients you might find on a label that could be causing damage to your body. So only put back in the fridge or cupboard any food that does NOT include any of the ingredients on this list.

After taking an inventory of all the foods that could be causing damage to your body, you can make the choice to either throw them away or put them back. This will give you an idea as to what extent your existing diet is less than ideal, which can really put your present eating habits into perspective. You may find that taking a picture of the exercise will serve as a healthy reminder the next time you visit the grocery store. Check out my podcast, "Your Life Is Nonnegotiable," where I visit my clients' homes and rummage through their cupboards and fridges, helping them identify the toxic chemicals lurking in the foods they are feeding their families.

Food ingredients to be avoided are as follows:

- Sodium nitrate

- Sulfites

- Azodicarbonamide

- Propyl gallate

- BHA/BHT

- Propylene glycol

- Butane

- Monosodium glutamate (MSG)
- Disodium inosinate
- Disodium guanylate
- Enriched flour
- Recombinant bovine growth hormone (rBGH)
- Refined vegetable oil
- Sodium benzoate
- Brominated vegetable oil
- Carrageenan
- Polysorbate
- Carnauba wax
- Magnesium sulfate
- Paraben
- Sodium carboxymethyl cellulose
- Aluminum
- Saccharin
- Aspartame
- High-fructose corn syrup
- Acesulfame potassium
- Sucralose
- Agave nectar
- Bleached starch
- Tert butylhydroquinone
- Red #40

- Blue #1

- Blue #2

- Citrus red #2

- Green #3

- Yellow #5

- Yellow #6

- Red #2

- Red #3

- Caramel coloring

- Brown HT

- Orange B

- Bixin

- Norbixin

- Annatto

SETTING YOU UP FOR SUCCESS

Why "Eat Less, Move More" Is a Big Fat Lie!

This is one of the most commonly made assertions, and also misconceptions, about weight loss. Everyone has heard someone say "Eat less, move more." Well, it's not quite that simple, to say the least. If nutrition were that simple, then no one would ever encounter any problems.

In reality, body composition, exercise, hormones, genetics, your microbiome, and food quality and composition all play a huge role. Contrary to popular belief, there is only a small correlation between weight loss and calories. The entire calorie concept is rather flawed. Few of us question how this concept came into being, but there is an intriguing tale to be told here.

Creation of Calories

The invention and discovery of the calorie concept are often associated with French chemist Nicolas Clément, as he first documented the concept in 1824. Since then, it has become central to the nutritional approach of millions of people.

Yet despite the cultural prominence of calories, dissenting voices have frequently questioned their actual value. James Hamblin, MD, wrote a pointed article in *The Atlantic* entitled, "Forget Calories," in which the nutritional correspondent recommended people focus on the actual food that they eat rather than the dated concept of calories.

A calorie is literally a unit of energy. It is defined as the amount of energy needed to raise the temperature of one gram of water by one degree Celsius at a pressure of one atmosphere. It was measured in the nineteenth century by burning food into ash, and thus is more about how much energy is required to induce food to disintegrate rather than the energy content of the food itself.

Different Bodies, Different Outcomes

However, as we will continually learn throughout this book, everyone's body is different. Each person will require a different level of energy in order to break down food. This is never factored into the so-called calorie count. Our individual gut microbiome (we will be explaining this concept and talking more about the microbiome as the book unfolds, so don't worry if you're not familiar with this at present) has a massive influence over how our bodies work, and this renders a simple, averaged-out measure of calories rather redundant.

Another problem is that when you attempt to count calories, your body will adjust. Creating a calorie deficit can have some impact, but at this point, the body will enter into a process of homeostasis. This simply refers to the tendency of biological organisms to auto-regulate and maintain their internal environment in a stable state. In other words, things change in order to adapt to the new climate.

So when your body senses that you're only giving it 1,500 calories per day instead of 2,000, it simply decides that it is now only necessary to burn 1,500 calories. This means that you're often achieving very little over the long term with calorie counting. Far more effective is cajoling the body into a state of ketosis, which we'll talk about later on.

Here is another common problem: People often engage in a period of dieting and reach their weight loss goal. Great! At that point, all of their discipline about eating goes out the window. They think they can eat whatever they want again. But their body has now adjusted to receiving fewer calories, so as soon as they revert to their old level of food intake . . . the weight gradually creeps back on. Sound familiar?

Why Hormones Matter

Hormones play a significant role in the overall body weight picture, particularly insulin. Insulin is a fat-storing hormone and will be mentioned several times throughout this book. Insulin spikes to counteract the glucose in our bloodstream when we consume foods high in carbohydrates or sugar. As a result of this, over time, it is possible for the body to become insulin resistant, which leads to obesity, weight gain, and type 2 diabetes, among other conditions.

So, with this in mind, calories are not the most important factor in weight loss and overall health, compared to the energy differential created between what we eat and later burn. This is particularly influenced by the actual food that we consume and how it interacts with our hormones.

The Exercise Issue

Exercise also has a major influence on the way our bodies operate. I'm sure you're aware that we all have a different body metabolism, and the rate of this metabolism can be significantly impacted by our level of physical activity. We all know that physical activity is important, yet many myths tend to circulate about the best way to exercise in order to help the body.

Ultimately, exercise is energy out. Exercise enables us to burn up the energy that we derive from food. However, it's also important to understand that there is such a thing as over-exercising. This seems like a contradiction in terms, as we tend to believe that the more exercise we engage in, the better it is for the body.

However, if you are consuming a regular amount of food—and not the vast quantities that an elite athlete eats, for example—then as soon as you punish the body with excessive degrees of exercise, it will panic and cling to the energy that you've accumulated via food rather than burning it off. You may also experience some other symptoms that are far from desirable. Adrenal fatigue, weight gain, sleep deprivation, and increased body fat are all possible if you exercise too much.

This is because you wreak havoc with your hormones if you exercise too much. If you fail to give your body the rest that it needs in order to function properly, then it can be negatively impacted; hence the term *adrenal fatigue*. When the body suffers from this condition, adrenal glands become depleted due to their producing insufficient stress hormones, including cortisol.

Moderation in All Things

So training in moderation is undoubtedly a positive thing, as this will be in balance with your body's internal systems. But how much is too much and how much is too little? Well, the first thing to address is that everyone's body will respond differently to exercise. It is advisable to exercise every day, but what constitutes exercise can actually be something rather light. It can be nearly 20 minutes of stretching or yoga, or maybe a walking meditation.

It's important to remember that as little as 100 years ago, our bodies were in motion throughout the day, every day, 365 days a year. We were designed to hunt, gather, lift, pull, push, hike, walk, swim, run, tuck, craw, climb, and move our bodies in all ranges of motion. Today, we try to simulate the varied forms of motion using HIIT training, CrossFit, marathons, triathlons, weight training, Zumba, yoga, Pilates, and so much more. Always listen to your body. This is always one of my biggest challenges with my clients. Either they don't train enough because they are afraid of overdoing it, or they over-train their bodies as they perceive that the only way to weight loss is to burn as many calories as possible. Your body can handle a lot more than you think it can, but may not need the excessive, aggressive attacks that we inflict upon it.

We should draw a distinction between exercise and training. We can consider training to be more intense, although it is still possible to overtrain. Intensity and duration are key here, with experts now believing that oxidative stress is beneficial in small amounts.

Oxidative stress has quite a fancy and complex medical definition. Merriam-Webster defines it as "physiological stress on the body that is caused by the cumulative damage done by free radicals inadequately neutralized by antioxidants and that is held to be associated with aging."When experienced excessively, oxidative stress can be damaging, but in moderation it can have positive impacts.

When the body responds to stress, it prepares itself for the possibility of injury or infection. Central to this process is the production of extra chemicals that help regulate the immune system. This provides a temporary defensive boost and has been corroborated by animal studies from Harvard University. So the process of oxidative stress prompts our bodies to become both stronger and younger as they benefit from an increase in antioxidants.

The good news is that most forms of exercise create some form of oxidative stress, effectively meaning that they are all beneficial for our bodies. This is one of the fundamental reasons that exercise tends to make us healthier. Your body is slightly weakened in the aftermath; you go through a recovery period and gradually become more resistant to additional oxidative stress workload.

Limited Capacity

However, your body does have a limited capacity to increase its antioxidants in order to control free radicals (these are atoms or groups of atoms with an odd number of electrons, which can be formed when oxygen interacts with certain molecules). Marathon running can simply be too much for many people's bodies, meaning that they fail to derive any benefit from it, and it even ultimately damages their anatomy.

This doesn't mean that cardio work involving endurance is worthless. Far from it. But such forms of exercise should be done in moderation in order to allow the body time to recover. They can instead be combined with restorative workouts, such as Pilates, yoga, stretching, walking meditations, power walking, Tai Chi, light strength training, and stationary bike cycling.

Concentrating on these restorative techniques during the six-week program is particularly recommended, and I will reiterate my exercise recommendations later in this text. But you should absolutely give your body a chance to heal, your hormones the opportunity to rest, and your adrenals a few moments to catch up while engaging in a program of training and exercise.

Master Your Metabolism

One of the key concepts that we will explore in this book is that of ketosis, which is central to weight loss.

Before discussing this, it's important to understand that the body is able to use three separate forms of fuel for energy:

- Glucose, or sugar

- Ketones

- Muscle

The body will always burn what is most readily available. For almost all people, this will be glucose. Every time you consume sugar and carbs they are converted and stored as both glucose and glycogen. Glucose is the easiest form of energy for our bodies to use, so naturally it will be burned before anything else if you provide it to your body.

But we don't want that. We want to convert our bodies into fat burners. Becoming a fat-burning machine may sound trendy and might land you on the cover of *Shape* magazine; however, it's important to understand that our bodies thrive in the fat-burning state of ketosis. Our machines were primitively designed to utilize fat as our primary fuel source. One way to achieve this is to adopt a ketogenic diet. Although a ketogenic diet is very fashionable, I'm not necessarily recommending it in this book, as it is not always suitable for everyone. We are all different.

Easing into Ketosis

Instead, I advocate a modified eating plan that will ease your body into ketosis allied with a plan of intermittent fasting. Combining the two will soon have your body burning fat, and that is exactly what we're looking for. These concepts might seem a bit scary and intimidating right now, but we're going to walk you through the science and show you how they will benefit your body, your health, and your life.

Central to the concept of ketosis is reducing the number of carbohydrates that you consume. I'm sure that you've encountered this concept at some point, as many approaches to diet and nutrition advocate this aspect of eating.

The main reason that we're going to be looking at this dietary concept is that consuming carbs tends to prevent entering the state of ketosis—although we all have a different ketogenic limit—as these carbohydrates are converted into sugar, and the body burns that first. We don't want that! We want the body to become a fat burner, so it's necessary to reduce—though not necessarily eliminate—carbs.

Keeping carbohydrate consumption low can also have a wide range of health benefits. Evidence indicates that low-carb diets can be used to treat type 2 diabetes, weight-loss resistance, neurological disorders like Alzheimer's and Parkinson's disease, epilepsy, chronic headaches, ADD, sleep disorders, autism, and even brain cancer.

This is not to say that we don't need carbohydrates. We do. We were designed to eat seasonally and locally where carbohydrates, fats, and proteins were available in cycles. You may have heard of trendy terms today such as *carb cycling* or *metabolic flexibility*, which basically mean that your body is designed to fluctuate between these energy sources as your body constantly adapts to the foods that are readily available during certain seasons and locations of the world at any given time. But one rule of thumb is a must. Your carbs, fats, and proteins must come in the form of whole foods grown naturally from the ground or from animals that roam freely, eating the foods their bodies were designed to consume. Any food with a label on it is likely harmful. So do your research on processed foods, and if you have to buy labeled food, choose the ones with the fewest ingredients as possible. Consult my podcast, "Your Life Is Nonnegotiable," for more education on this topic.

Remember, this is a six-week program. I'm not about to ask you to stick to it resolutely for the rest of your life. Far from it. But you might want to take the basic principles on board and use this to inform your eating habits and lifestyle going forward.

Furthermore, we're going to hook you up with a brilliant community and support group, which will help make the transition that much easier. We're all about helping you transition steadily if that's what you want and need. This program and lifestyle will fit around your needs rather than dictating what you need to do.

Water and Hydration

Probably the most neglected aspect of health is hydration. This really is a chronic problem in our society. So many of us drink large amounts of caffeinated drinks and soda, neither of which are doing anything for our state of hydration. And hydration really is important in terms of overall health, and specifically weight loss.

Water has a profound effect on cellular function, hormonal regulation, digestion, and gut health. There really is no excuse for not ensuring that you are properly hydrated, and this is really something that you should maintain over the long term. While not everything that you will be doing during this six-week process should be considered permanent, ensuring that you are properly hydrated should absolutely be part of your everyday life.

Chronic Dehydration

Drinking water first thing in the morning is a habit that you should instantly adopt in your life. Get yourself on good hydration footing from the very beginning of your day. Drinking more water will prevent you from being part of the 75 percent of people in Western society deemed to be chronically dehydrated. And, of course, this condition has some serious side effects.

First, those who are chronically dehydrated will face fat-loss and weight-loss resistance. Chronic dehydration slows down the body's metabolism, as your body naturally requires a certain quantity of water in order to engage in metabolic processing. Dehydration also makes it hard for our bodies to utilize energy as fuel, meaning that ketosis is effectively impossible.

Chronic dehydration can also contribute to digestive problems, as hydration is essential for every bodily function. Bloating and water retention can also result because when the body perceives itself to be lacking in water it deems this to be an extremely serious attack, and it then concludes that it must hold on to what energy, weight, and sustenance it already has.

People who do not drink enough water often feel bloated and puffy, which can then make them restrict their water intake. This only compounds the situation. Meanwhile, their bodies are retaining too much water because they're not getting enough hydration. Additional signs of chronic dehydration include brain fog, headaches, depression, low blood pressure, and inability to focus.

You should be aiming to drink between 75 and 100 ounces of water every day. Start planning to drink more water starting now, right as you're reading this. This is something you can do to help your body immediately. There really is no excuse for not ensuring that you are properly hydrated. Yes, kicking the soda or coffee habit can be tricky, but these beverages are doing far more harm than good.

So we're going to get into this program in a lot more detail—all the science behind it and all the benefits that you will ultimately garner from it. But first of all, I'm going to tell you my story and how I ended up where I am today.

Chapter One

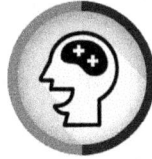

My Story

I NEVER TOOK MY HEALTH SERIOUSLY UNTIL I WAS IN MY MIDTWENTIES. You know how it is when you're young and you think you can just sail through life without anything impacting you. Well, for a long time, I was kidding myself, and it was only going through some of my more negative life experiences that made me truly understand how important health and well-being really are.

Now I am ecstatic with where I am in life today. I feel extremely happy about what I have been able to achieve and the state of my body, health, and lifestyle. Yay for me! (*Pats own back*) But this sense of stability and satisfaction didn't come easily.

In my younger years, I definitely wasn't the person I am today. It is my story, my experience, that has inspired me to want to help others, and which underpins everything I do today. And I firmly believe that others can learn from my experience.

My Early Years

Between the ages of 19 and 23, I put on a lot of weight. And I mean a *lot*. I was eating Kraft dinners, KFC; I was having bacon-butter sandwiches for supper. My diet was pretty terrible. I was drinking and smoking too much. Sounds like fun, right?

It wasn't fun! I was really struggling with who I was and with the things that had happened to me, and I was having a hard time pulling myself out of the mental hole that I was in. I was really depressed. I was in debt. In fact, I was suicidal. I had attempted suicide three times. Things were about as low as they could go for me.

This cycle worsened as I attempted to anesthetize myself against these feelings. I think I realized what I was doing at the time, and that it was counterproductive, but I didn't know any other way to cope with my situation other than to drink, smoke, party, and generally attempt to bury my negative thoughts in an alcoholic haze. Guess what? It didn't work!

Turning the Tide

Because of my sink-or-swim mentality, I decided to pick up the pieces and go back to start a new life in Montreal, my hometown. I had been in Ottawa for six years prior to that. When I got back, I started paying a little more attention to my health. I started eating better. I started walking on a treadmill every day for 45 minutes while listening to self-help gurus, like Tony Robbins, and all sorts of other fascinating and informative people.

So I decided to change my diet and make a concerted effort to lose weight. This was partly for health and appearance reasons, but also due to the fact that I simply felt terrible about myself. I was determined to change my life, but a lack of education and knowledge was also an issue at this time.

Based on my relatively minimal understanding, I began consuming a diet consisting of three solid meals every day. Knowing what I know today, I would have done things completely differently.

Nonetheless, I slowly but surely started to pull myself out of my mental hole. I lost 30 pounds. I was starting to feel better. I didn't understand nutrition to the degree that I do now, but I was beginning to take my health more seriously, I started to educate myself and read many books, and then I decided to get the appropriate certification in fitness and nutrition. Relying on a meal plan was not enough—I needed to understand more.

It took me quite some time to achieve positive results, but I was pretty pleased that I'd at least made some progress. However, around 12 months into attempting to craft the new me, I hit the infamous plateau. *Bang!* I hit that wall pretty hard!

I began to miss eating all of my favorite foods, and my motivation to continue my efforts seriously diminished. The natural outcome of that mindset was that I began to incorporate my favorite foods back into my life and diet once again.

My motivation for the gym had also begun to dwindle, and the reasons for this were quite obvious. I no longer experienced the results that were evident when I started, and there were also other underlying issues that were proving to be demotivating.

Hammer Blow

Then, one day, I went to visit my grandmother in the hospital. I would do this every month or so, but this particular visit was the most shocking to me, and it was truly one of the most impactful days of my life.

She had been sharing her hospital room with three other people, and the guy in the next bed started moaning, wailing, and making all sorts of crazy noises. I looked over, kind of giggling at my grandmother. I said, "Nan, what's the matter with him?"

At that moment, it wasn't what she said; it was the way she said it. I looked into her eyes, and her eyes darted back at me. They were piercing, and tears welled up in her eyes as she said, "Sherry, he never stops. He never stops." She was so frustrated. She was so aggravated. She was so tired. She was afraid. She was lonely. You could feel so much emotion in that one sentence.

It forever changed my life. As I looked around the room—and although the room was decent—I could see it definitely needed an upgrade. The walls were a little dingy, the windows weren't particularly clean, the lighting flickered, and there was a pretty pungent smell. You could smell medications. You could smell bedpans. You could just smell hospital.

Then I suddenly realized that because my grandmother had suffered a stroke and was paralyzed from the left side down, she was completely stranded in her hospital bed. And it became her jail cell. This was her jail cell for the last six years of her life. She couldn't move when she wanted. She couldn't go to the bathroom when she wanted. She couldn't even reach for a magazine beside her if she wanted one, because she couldn't move from the left side down.

This is how she spent her last six years. When I left that day, I decided right then and there that my health was nonnegotiable. I would do absolutely everything in my power to be as fit and healthy as I could possibly be.

The Road Ahead

From then on, I focused on education. I continued to acquire additional certifications, took more university courses, bought a huge amount of books and online courses, and attended workshops and conferences, and I've basically been obsessed with learning everything that there is to know about the human anatomy.

I don't want what happened to my grandmother to happen to me. I don't want to be in that old-age home. I don't want to be in pain. I don't want to live every day with chronic hip pain, neck pain, arthritis, or Alzheimer's, or not be able to remember my own name. I watched someone die of ALS—amyotrophic lateral sclerosis, a horrible condition that affects nerve cells in the brain and spinal cord—which basically robbed her of her life and resulted in a very slow and painful death.

I made a firm pact with myself that I would work aggressively to make my health nonnegotiable.

However, although I really wanted to progress further at this point, I also felt hugely confused and conflicted. There was a vast amount of information out there, and I felt conflicted by which direction to turn. I didn't know what advice to follow, and meanwhile, any positive results had completely dried up. This was naturally reducing my motivation.

Luckily, at this point I decided to hire a personal trainer, figuring that a professional could help me get back on the right track. This was instrumental in my progression, as I learned a great deal about weight training thanks to this decision. And sure enough, I began to see results. The more weight training I did, the more evident the results were. I began to think that I could acquire the same arms as Jennifer Aniston after all!

As I became more confident in my ability to weight train, I managed to win second prize in a transformation contest at the gym I attended. My body was really beginning to rip up now, and I felt better than ever. I could both feel and see my muscles developing, and I felt pretty pleased with my progress.

But there was a lot more to come.

The Fire Burns

At this time, I was asked whether or not I was interested in enrolling in a fitness and certification program, with the aim of becoming professionally qualified in the subject. I'm very glad to say that I jumped at the chance, and this really changed my entire mentality and outlook. A fire was lit inside me from this point, and I became extremely passionate about learning everything possible about the body, the mind, stress, sleep, hormones—effectively everything that goes together to constitute our well-being and health.

I learned as much as I possibly could, but this is very much an ongoing process. The passion for health and well-being has stayed with me ever since, and I still spend two to three hours every day studying the subject. I am continually researching the latest science, listening to podcasts, checking out the latest audiobooks, and generally keeping abreast of developments in health understanding and practice. You name it—I have studied it. I am a true biohacker!

So my passion eventually morphed into my career, and I began to help my peeps get educated on their minds, bodies, and emotions. This has become a critical and highly valued part of my personal journey, which has continued over the last decade.

Reaching People

Although I had come a long way by this point, and I was proud of what I had accomplished, I still encountered a new problem. I began to notice that there was somewhat of a disconnect between my clients and myself.

While I was hugely passionate about understanding the subject of health in depth, my clients were consumed only with the ultimate results of their efforts. They wanted to know when, where, and how these results would manifest on their bodies. It became clear to me that my clients were often stressed and overwhelmed by the challenges in their lives, and the extra learning and studying associated with understanding their bodies were simply too much for them to take on.

So it was necessary for me to come up with a solution that would enable my clients to achieve their goals and also fit their lifestyles. I wanted the people involved with the program to truly appreciate why I was creating certain habits, standards, and foundations of behavior for them in their lives. I wanted them to then take the next step and truly understand where they wanted to go with their bodies, health, and well-being goals in the future.

Understanding Health

This goes beyond mere aesthetics and shedding a few pounds, and enters an entirely holistic field of overall wellness. Rather than merely looking better, I wanted people to really *feel* better and understand diverse aspects of wellness. I wanted the program to be far more about health as a form of disease prevention, with the overall approach focused on mental clarity, removing anxiety, depression, and fears, and delivering a truly holistic approach to general well-being. Easier said than done, but it is possible!

As I mentioned previously, this is all about health at the cellular level. We all obviously tend to look at the external as an indicator of our well-being, but really the building blocks of health are internal. When these foundations evolve into a healthy state and are then maintained, our lives simply become a lot richer and more enjoyable.

But in order for my clients to understand this, it became obvious to me that I needed to condense the information into bite-size pieces. The bare bones and core of the program needed to be digestible, freeing participants from the need to concern themselves with deep scientific concepts.

Creating Our Community

From this initial seed of an idea, I began to create an online course at www.myhealthisnonnegotiable.com, and now this book. I am extremely enthusiastic about the course and the fantastic team of people I have been able to assemble. They are all hugely motivated to understand the body so that they REALLY, REALLY GET IT!

The course and the content of this book provide a powerful template for behavior. It will help you to eat and move your body in the way that it was actually designed to eat and move, based on state-of-the-art scientific research. The importance of support was also considered during this process, and an amazing community was created that goes well beyond the diktats of a mere piece of paper that tells you what to do and what to avoid.

While changing your habits for a short time can be relatively easy, it is also easy to slide back into damaging old behaviors. So we really believe that the community and support group that we have built up at www.myhealthisnonnegotiable.com is absolutely invaluable.

With this program, I have taken the tens of thousands of hours of research that I have engaged in over the years and condensed it into an amazing, easily digestible package. I have particularly focused on delivering small chunks of information that can be easily under-stood by clients on a daily basis.

We also provide mastermind groups, Facebook groups, and personal one-on-one chats in order to ensure that everyone has a fun experience. Because improving your health shouldn't be a chore, it should be fun! Right?

Your Health Is Nonnegotiable

This book is inspired by the first line of a celebration and mantra that we have created in order to outline the lifestyle that we help build for people. My health is nonnegotiable. Repeat that. My health is nonnegotiable.

> I am taking chaos and confusion out of my life and creating control and certainty in my soul.
>
> I am learning how to biohack my mind, my hormones, and my body to a guiltless freedom.
>
> I understand that this body was the only asset I was ever given.
>
> And because today is the first day of the rest of my life, I'm going to embrace this journey.
>
> This new, healthy journey.
>
> One step at a time.
>
> And for this, I am so excited.

So let's get into it—it's time for you to take control of your health.

Chapter Two

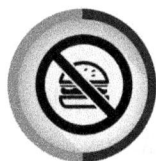

FASTING

THE GOAL THIS WEEK (WEEK ONE):

WE HAVE THREE GOALS FOR THIS WEEK:

1. To help you dramatically reduce sugar in your body.

2. To help you reduce the harmful vegetable oils that are present in almost all processed and restaurant foods.

3. To help you determine a fasting protocol—increase the window of time that you don't eat, and shorten the window of time that you do eat.

BEFORE WE START, I WANT TO EMPHASIZE THAT THESE ARE *YOUR* SIX WEEKS. You make all the decisions here. What we are offering you in this book is guidance based on the science of how the body was designed to survive. You must determine what is best for you while you experiment with your body.

In our Six-Week Transformation Program, we coach our members to start their programs with a fasting protocol for a few specific reasons.

Our first goal is to reduce the intake of sugar in the body. This will help to reduce the production of insulin, not to mention assisting with the regulation of other hormones as well.

Our second goal is to reduce harmful vegetable oils. This will help to rid your body of those horrible substances that are causing a hot mess within all your major systems.

Finally, our third goal is to help you create a fasting protocol that you can experiment with by increasing your fasting windows and decreasing your feeding windows. (Note: we are not talking about calorie reduction, but rather shifting the times when you fuel the body.)

Your Steps To Success

Adhering to a few of the following simple steps can help you propel your way to creating effective routines to kick-start your health. You can access the "Nonnegotiable Workbook" in order to help you personalize these steps in a fun and colorful way: www.myhealthis-nonnegotiable.com/workbook.

Step 1: Determine your feeding and fasting windows.

Step 2: Determine your resting metabolic rate.

Step 3: Determine what time of day you *might* choose to eat your carbs.

Step 4: Determine how many meals you wish to have during the day.

Step 5: Decide your first fuels (fats and proteins), second fuels (carbs, if necessary), and third fuels (optional, but light); see the recommended recipes in *Your Health Is Nonnegotiable Cookbook.*

Top Ten Tips To Get You Started

Before we dive deep into the science of fasting, here are a few quick tips to help you experiment with this concept. Reading the science aspect behind fasting will increase your confidence once you establish a true appreciation of the benefits. So here are some tips that I will expand on as the chapter unfolds:

1. Listen to your body.

2. Plan ahead for success.

3. Preparation is key.

4. Have a backup plan.

5. Don't talk to friends or family about fasting just yet.

6. Participate in our online community.

7. Know yourself and listen to your instincts.

8. Limit your carb window.

9. Exercise in a fasted state.

10. Don't compare yourself to others.

I'm sure that the concept of fasting is something that is very new to you and your lifestyle. It's something that we tend to associate with religious practice or a hunger strike. Let's face it—our modern culture doesn't involve a great deal of fasting! It does involve a great deal of unnecessary and unhealthy snacking, but fasting . . . not so much!

So let's get a better understanding of the goals we will set and why they are important.

GOAL ONE: Sugar Circulation

Our first goal is to reduce the sugar circulating around your system, which often emanates from a significant intake of carbohydrates. However, the approach that we are going to take to fasting, and the diet changes that you will make, will not represent a lifelong decision. I will not be pushing you into the trendy keto diet, but I am going to outline the science of ketosis and its benefits to your well-being for the short term. This is a concept that you might flirt with weekly, monthly, or annually. There are five main ways to fast. In fact, I created a short, free video on this topic where I dive into deeper detail, which you can find at www.myhealthisnonnegotiable.com/freevideos.

Our second goal is to drastically reduce your consumption of vegetable oils along with additional chemicals and preservatives found in processed and restaurant food. Every modern food product with a label almost inevitably contains vegetable oils, chemicals, and preservatives, but the good news is that there are quite a few new companies which are riding the "healthy, chemical-free" bandwagon. They are producing foods that don't include these unnecessary ingredients. However, be mindful of false, misleading packaging. These guys are very clever at masking harmful ingredients on food labeling. Go to the following link to find a free video I produced on food labels and how big businesses disguise these chemicals: www.myhealthisnonnegotible.com/freevideos.

Our third goal is to increase your fasting windows and decrease your feeding windows. Now! Before you freak out, take a breath . . . ah . . . that's better! You're totally in charge of this decision. You decide what is best for you and your lifestyle.

Before you digest all the science, I'm going to guide you through a step-by-step fasting process. In order to do this, I'm going to use some useful tips and tricks so that you can steadily adjust to your fasting experiment. We've mapped out a beautiful way to help you organize, plan, and be accountable for achieving the goals you set for yourself, in the form of a workbook. Match the tips with the science shared below, and then create your plan in the workbook. You can find the workbook at: www.myhealthisnonnegotiable.com/workbook.

Step 1: Defining Your Feeding And Fasting Windows

Fasting may sound like a drastic process, but few of us are actually aware of the definition of the word itself. Fasting is simply the distance of time between two meals. As we go through the science, you will learn more about why increasing your fasting hours and decreasing your feeding windows will help regulate your hormones, improve the quality of your sleep, and, believe it or not, actually give you more energy.

I should also emphasize that there are various ways of fasting (see your free video as mentioned above), but for now, we're just going to look at intermittent fasting. I want to remind you that you are in complete control of this process. You set your own fasting hours and do what suits you, your lifestyle, your family, and your body. This plan must be structured so that it is appropriate for your needs. That is the most important thing.

I encourage people to start off easily and then ease their way into increasing their fasting hours as they become more comfortable. You could start with a 12-hour fast, which you are probably doing already! We usually try to stop eating before bed, and it's common to go for 12 hours without eating again. Say, from 8 p.m. to 8 a.m. So to begin with a 12-hour window shouldn't be too difficult to tackle. I will then encourage you to steadily increase this period as you become more comfortable with the concept and process.

Step 2: Resting Metabolic Rate

The second important step is to capture your resting metabolic rate; this is the level of caloric burn your body requires on a daily basis in order to keep all bodily functions . . . well . . . functioning. This can be recorded with a smartwatch, or an approximate calculator can be found by Googling "resting metabolic rate calculator." The smartwatch reading will provide a better indication, although it is still not 100 percent accurate. But, either way, you will have a good idea of what your body is burning without exercise and will be in a better position to prepare yourself to lose fat.

It is important to capture this figure, as it will provide you with a useful guide of how much food is needed to sustain you on a daily basis if you do absolutely nothing, and how much food your body will burn off in its daily functioning.

Step 3: Carb Munching

The good news for those of you who particularly enjoy carbs is that we are not going to eliminate them completely during this week. Our third step is to reduce your overall carb intake, but you can still choose to eat some carbohydrates during this seven-day period. Yes, I encourage you to decrease your overall carb load, but I don't want you to put yourself through massive and needless discomfort. It should be noted that it is encouraged to work yourself into a state of ketosis by eventually eliminating carbs temporarily. We want you to be able to "listen" to your body and the signs and signals it can send you when foods don't agree with your system. This will all be further explained as we go. But . . . baby steps.

If you are physically and mentally addicted to carbs (which you may not fully realize), then you might experience some symptoms that represent what is sometimes referred to as the "keto flu"; this is simply your body detoxing from sugar and unraveling its addiction to all forms of sugar. But we will go into that in more detail later in the chapter. Caution: if you are diabetic, or if you're on medication, you must do your research or consult your doctor before making drastic changes to your diet.

Keep in mind, many people believe that they follow a healthy diet, but if your food comes from a bag, box, or a bottle, more than likely, sugar has been added. Many people eat more fruit than their bodies were designed for, which of course can also be very high in sugar.

If your intention is to include carbs as part of your diet during the fasting period, you should choose a time of day that you're allowed to eat them. This should be when you are most active, so the afternoon, when you're up and about, is probably the best time to consume carbohydrates. Penciling in a window around 3–6 p.m. is advisable.

Step 4: Meal Choices

The fourth step that you should undertake before beginning the fasting process is considering how many meals you are going to consume each day. Most people will likely maintain their three meals a day while cutting out the snacks. You'll find as you increase your fasting windows you will go down to two or even one meal a day.

There will be much more information later on in this chapter about why eating less, moving more, and grazing on food several times per day are simply messages that we've been told repeatedly over the last half-century. These ideas are neither entirely accurate nor beneficial.

Step 5: Finalizing Fuels

You also need to make a decision over the three "fuels" that you will put in your body. I refer to these feeding times as fuels because there are times when you literally need to fuel your body with what it needs to get through the day. Your fuel is simply the nourishment that your body requires in order to be at its peak performance. I believe that there are times to eat and enjoy our food, savor the flavors, and enjoy the textures and the smells, especially when we have chosen to be social and connect with other people. In my opinion, this should constitute 20 percent of your feeding time. Most of the time the goal is to nourish your body from sunrise to sunset with the proper nutrients it needs to function at its peak performance. This should effectively occur 80 percent of the time.

My personal methodology is that, from Monday to a certain point in time on the weekend, I eat to nourish my body the way it was designed to eat, and then, at certain chosen times, I eat for the pleasure of eating. You don't have to follow this, but it provides you with a possible template for your own approach.

So you will decide the time for your first fuel, which should be comprised of healthy fats and protein. Your second fuel can incorporate some carbohydrates, but I recommend steering away from bread, pasta, rice, and all starchy foods. Instead, choose healthier carbs such as low glycemic fruits and berries. Try to limit your carb intake as much as possible at this time, as incorporating carbs will prevent your body from getting into a state of ketosis.

If you choose to have a third meal, this will likely be around supper time, and I recommend having a light meal, focusing primarily on fats and proteins.

Step 6: Training Schedule

The final step that you should take in this fasting process is to design a suitable training schedule for yourself. It's important to remember that if this is your first time experimenting with fasting and carb-cutting, you may experience some withdrawal symptoms. You can still work out safely, but you should listen to your body at all times and certainly not overdo it if you are struggling with what is often referred to as carb flu. This is a short period during which your body reacts against the removal of its usual carb load and you experience headaches, brain fog, tiredness, and other undesirable symptoms. It does get better pretty quickly, though, and we'll discuss the reasons why this happens later on.

At first, I can guarantee that you will feel fatigued and experience low energy. You will wonder if working out is a good idea while fasting. Once your body is more fat-adapted, and you have passed the keto flu, you will feel a lot more energized. Working out will feel better the more that you practice and the stronger you get. If you have not been working out for a while and you are jumping back on the workout train, then listen to your body and start off with light to moderate workouts. If you feel dizzy and noxious, don't panic; just stop and lie on your back with all of your limbs stretched out. Do not cross or bend your limbs. Wait for your heart rate to fall back to resting (under 100 bpm). Breathe deeply. Inhale through the nose and exhale through the mouth. The dizziness and nausea will pass within 10–15 minutes. Please consult a professional health practitioner if you are concerned.

Now: fasting is not only perfectly safe, it's also very natural for the body. For tens of thousands of years, our bodies endured both feasts and famines. Our bodies survived in a world that was seasonal and cyclical. This is normal. However, for your entire existence on this planet, you've probably ingested processed foods, and this has potentially altered your anatomical chemistry. So it's important to take some precautions when fasting. Your body has become accustomed to one way of being, and you now have to cajole it into another way of being.

With this in mind, in this next section, I'm going to cover my top tips for practicing fasting safely.

Tip 1: Listen To Your Body

Your body will speak volumes if you just listen to it. Everyone's body is different, and we're all dealing with different issues and life experiences. For example, you may be taking medication or dealing with a particular illness. Our goal here is not to put you through massive amounts of discomfort. Although it can be normal to go through some periods where you feel a little off-color when undertaking this program, you must nonetheless react to symptoms that intuitively feel off course. We have a wonderful team in our Six-Week Transformation Program, so if you are at all nervous about going through this experience alone, reach out to us for support at www.yourhealthisnonnegotiable.com/support.

I should also mention that you shouldn't be fasting at all if you are pregnant, breastfeeding, elderly, or a child/adolescent. If you do encounter any severe symptoms that you can't cope with, there is a simple solution: eat! You can always try to fast again the next day.

Tip 2: Plan Ahead For Success

When you initially embark on this new program, the first couple of days, and even weeks, are an adjustment period. It's imperative that you plan ahead for success! I usually recommend Sunday mornings for this process, as in most homes that's the quietest time to head into the kitchen to prep your food for the week. This is a great opportunity to set goals, and plan your eating habits around your work/family schedule for the week ahead.

If you're part of our online program, your knowledgeable coaches will help you design your 42-day plan. They will support you with your choice of meals, your preparation and eating schedule, and other facets of your lifestyle, in order to ensure that you have the appropriate knowledge to set you up for success.

Tip 3: Preparation Is Key

Although nutrients begin to dissipate the moment that fruits and vegetables are pulled from their stems or roots, and even more so once they are chopped, I still like to promote prepping salads and such in advance because I believe the value of being well-prepared for your week and ready to fight those hunger cravings far outweighs the nutrient deficiency.

There are contradictory opinions on this, but in my program, I promote a healthy green smoothie or green powdered supplement in the morning, in order to properly nourish your body and your gut in a hydrated form on an empty stomach. I believe we already have an uphill battle when it comes to acquiring satisfactory nourishment from foods. We have leaky guts, we have chemicals in our food, we have saturated soils, we have the oxidation of plants once they are picked from the ground, we have reduced hydrochloric acid in our stomachs. And on and on it goes!

So I suggest that you prepare all of your meals so that they're ready in a pinch. You should have meals on hand in the fridge, your office, and in your car at all times. You can then have continual access to nutritious, healthy food when you need it most.

Tip 4: Have A Backup Plan

Not everything in life works out as planned. Boy, don't we know it! I strongly encourage you to KNOW and prepare your backup plan for both fitness and nutrition. Always know the alternatives to fitness when your workout gets bumped, and always have some spare healthy fats on hand for when your meals get delayed or you get that unexpected invitation to have lunch with a friend.

In terms of the training program, an online course is available to ensure that you never miss a workout, with highly interactive virtual classes that you can do from home. A truckload of prerecorded workouts is also available to ensure that you need never miss your daily dose of training.

Tip 5: Don't Talk To Friends
And Family About Fasting Just Yet

Once you have gone through this book, it is perfectly natural to become evangelical about the subject of health. I have been there myself! Although you may have the best intentions, it is not particularly wise to begin lecturing your family and friends on the subject. You will experience a great deal of opposition if you attempt this, as people are naturally resistant to things that they know little about, particularly if they represent a paradigm shift in their thinking. You may have heard this referred to as *cognitive dissonance.*

Get yourself educated first, and with that education will come renewed confidence. At that point, you can begin to share your informed understanding with those who are close to you, if you choose to do so. But you should always be prepared for some opposition and skepticism. Sorry, that's just the way of the world! You can lead someone to water, but you can't make him drink.

Tip 6: Participate In
Our Online Community

You don't have to do this alone! You don't have to keep your new-found enthusiasm under lock and key! You might instead decide to join our Six-Week Transformation Program online. Our online community is one of the aspects of the transformation of which I'm the proudest. I absolutely urge you to get involved. You will meet exceptional people in that community with whom you will get the opportunity to share your day-to-day experience. They are going through or have gone through your same journey.

Tip 7: Know Yourself
And Follow Your Instincts

The beauty of this program is that it is designed and created by you. Sure, you are using our guidance as a tool to create and design your new style of living. But you create all the rules. You redefine your lifestyle. You redefine the way you eat, you redefine the way you move your body—you are in complete control. Do not allow yourself to be influenced by other opinions; evaluate the knowledge you are receiving, do your own research, and come to your own conclusions as to what will suit you and your lifestyle best.

If you like to really throw yourself into something, and it has to be either all or nothing, then this is absolutely the right approach for you. But if you're a person who prefers gradual change, choose that path. There is no right or wrong way to do things; there is only the right way for you.

Tip 8: Limit Your Carb Window

There is no doubt that Western people in particular consume too many carbs. This is problematic not only for our collective health, but also for the six-week program. Heavy carbohydrate consumption inevitably leads to increased blood sugar, which means that our bodies end up burning sugar. If you're looking to burn more fat and use fat as an energy fuel source, then reducing your intake of carbs with a high glycemic index would be a great start.

So what I recommend during the program is to limit the window of time during which you consume carbohydrates. You don't have to phase carbs out completely. Instead, look to limit the amount you eat and also create a narrow window for your carb consumption. The principle will help you burn more fat, and it will make a big difference in how your body reacts and responds to the program.

It should also be noted that vegetables, greens, and low-glycemic foods should be favored sources of carbohydrates. You should consult with a medical practitioner if you are diabetic, as it's obviously particularly important for those dealing with diabetes to consume a suitably balanced diet.

Tip 9: Exercise In A Fasted State

One of the key things to bear in mind with your workout regime is that exercising in a fasted state is hugely beneficial. If your blood glucose level is low, you're more likely to be in ketosis and in a fat-burning state. It is also advisable to steer away from frequent high-intensity workouts all the time, as these are not beneficial for your goals. Be sure to incorporate a cross-training program that includes restorative training as well as fat-burning endurance training. Too much of anything is never good. So vary your workouts and give your body an opportunity to repair itself with proper rest periods. Don't make this a guessing game. Contact our professionals at www.myhealthisnon-negotiable.com for proper professional guidance.

You need to be training at a fat-burning heart rate. If you would like to watch a free, short training video where I discuss the five different levels of heart rate, please visit www.myhealthisnonnegotiable.com/freevideos.

Tip 10: Don't Compare Yourself To Others

Remember, this is your journey. You have to do things on your own terms and for yourself. Don't fall into the trap of comparing yourself to others. Definitely don't be hard on yourself. This program is a learning process, and it must match your lifestyle.

Everyone is different, and everyone's lifestyle is different. Your hormone production will be different from other people's. Your genetics and the makeup of your anatomy—every single aspect of you is different from other people.

People have different ways of reacting and adapting to this program, and your bodies will also react differently. So don't fall into the trap of unfairly comparing yourself, or your progress, to other people. Realize, understand, and accept that the journey is yours alone.

YOUR MORNING ROUTINE

Hydration

Next, I want to emphasize how important it is to establish a morning routine and stick to it. By beginning the day in the appropriate way, we kick-start our body into a positive state for the rest of the day. Getting into healthy habits at this time is absolutely essential to winning the rest of your day.

The first thing you should definitely do is hydrate, hydrate, hydrate! It is vital to ensure that you are properly hydrated from the moment that you wake up, and this is why I recommend keeping water by your bedside so that you can have a drink as soon as you're properly conscious. Ideally, you should use filtered water. I personally prefer the AquaTru system. In my private membership area I discuss all the products that I use personally.

Gratitude

It is imperative that you start your day on a positive frequency. I am religious about starting my day with positive, motivational, and inspirational messages that I receive via audiobooks or YouTube videos. I practice gratitude every single morning, and I appreciate everything I have accomplished and all that I have. It is so important to be conscious of the language you use to create your mental thoughts that then circulate in your brain. The law of attraction is extremely powerful. You can do anything and be anyone you wish to become with consistent hard work and effort. Do not engage in emails or social media or work until you have practiced gratitude and given yourself the gift of positive language.

Nutrients And Absorption

The next step is to get micronutrients into your body, and this can be achieved through your choice of a powdered green supplement added to water. I have always found an abundance of energy for the rest of my day as a result of this practice. The more hydration your body receives in the morning, the less fatigued you will feel in the afternoon. By ingesting a powdered green supplement of your choice first thing in the morning, you will hydrate and nourish your body and set yourself up for success.

Remember that your body is 65 percent water and requires hydration in order for your organs, muscles, brain, heart, and blood to function at their peak performance. As mentioned above, I believe you can increase your absorption of nutrients by choosing an organic, clean powdered green (plant-based) supplement. Be sure to do your homework on this one, or review the recommendations on my website.

I believe it is most beneficial to exercise first thing in the morning. Exercising on a fasted stomach can increase the fat you burn as fuel in your body, oxygenate your brain, and increase blood flow and circulation. You will also ignite powerful, positive hormones in your body that will serve you all day long.

Hunger Signals

One of the confusing things about our bodies is that we are sent the same hunger signal for three completely different reasons. The first of these is that we are actually hungry and need a big feed sooner rather than later! The second reason is that we are lacking nutrients in some form or another. The third is simple dehydration. It is also important to emphasize that hunger signals can be misleading, as they send off the exact same signal regardless of the reason they are occurring. So you may believe you're hungry for a big meal; however, what you actually are is dehydrated! All you need is a glass of water.

I suggest that the first step is to always have a big glass of water when you feel hungry. You should always begin the day with a glass of water, and this water should include some added minerals.

Step number two is to consider if you are well nourished at the time of hunger. If you have followed steps one and two and 20 minutes later are still hungry, then try eating a light meal.

So you can see that by imbibing water with nutrients at the very beginning of the day, you effectively eliminate the two misleading reasons for eating and ensure that your body will regulate itself successfully throughout the day.

However, it's also important not to overdo it with the nutrients, as too much can cause problems for your body. Signs that you are overdoing it include irritations, rashes, and bright yellow urine. Stick to the recommended dosage, and have a 12-hour gap between your two lumps of minerals for the day.

Recipe Ideas

We have compiled a list of recommended recipes to take you through each week of this program, which is provided in the cookbook. For week one, we share with you the most relevant recipes that will support your fasting experiment. In week two, we share recipes that will help you reduce inflammation in the body. In week three, we will show you how to nourish your gut by consuming probiotics, live cultures, fermented foods, and bone broth to nourish, replenish, and restore your microbiome (we will be coming to the topic of the microbiome in due course). We also share recipes for the cleansing and detox week, with some delicious juice and smoothie recipes.

The aim of your food intake during this 42-day period is to create new habits, so we have limited the recipes in order to minimize your choices, ensuring that you can concentrate on the process rather than agonize over food decisions. Everything you do going forward will come out of memory and habit. Once we have redefined your habits, you can begin to expand the types of food that you're eating and enjoy your usual variety.

Exercise Regimes

Before we get into the science of fasting, it's also important to go over your exercise program for the week. Exercise will be central to everything you do over these six weeks, and it absolutely goes hand in hand with nutrition. Now, I should start by saying that the first week is definitely not the week for high-intensity training. You need to be easy on your body as it begins to adapt to the program. You must also consider your lifestyle today as you begin the six-week process. If you're stressed, then your body will demand sugars and carbs (see the chapter on stress).

During this first week, you should embrace endurance running, breaking into a light jog or power walk. What you are looking for is long-distance fat-burning runs. Weight training will also be valuable during this period. Don't push yourself too hard, and don't do anything too extreme.

The Science Behind Fasting

Now we're going to move on to the science of fasting. This section will cover the following topics:

- What is fasting?

- The benefits of fasting

- Myths about fasting

- Different types of fasting

- Common symptoms that you may experience while fasting

There is a wide variety of interesting facts, citations, and scientific research included in this section, so I thoroughly recommend checking out the sources. At the end of this chapter, I will provide you with the story of one of my successful challengers because I feel this is so uplifting to hear. It's actually my favorite part of what I do!

The first important concept that I want to share with you in this section of the chapter is intermittent fasting. As soon as someone says the word *fasting* it conjures up extremely alarming thought processes! But this is just a conditioned response. In fact, when I began to research fasting and intermittent fasting, I discovered that there is strong scientific evidence which points to how good it is for the body and little to support the scaremongering. But more on that later.

By eating your food for the day within a shortened window, you achieve hunger regulation, increased fat loss, improved energy production, and superior gut health. Sounds like a no-brainer, right? Well, fasting shouldn't be seen as an absolutely critical tool for everyone, but it is certainly a process that benefits the vast majority of people, enabling them to develop a more metabolically flexible system. While a "metabolically flexible system" sounds like a bit of a mouthful, it is also something well worth aiming for. So let's go for it!

Hunger Hormones

Intermittent fasting enables you to take control of your hunger hormones. This will improve your insulin sensitivity, reduce the level of inflammation in your body, boost your everyday energy reserves, and enable you to lose weight without ever dieting. While all of these positive impacts on your biological systems are welcomed, that last one does sound particularly appealing. Whoever heard of someone losing weight without dieting? Well, it can be done!

Before going into the benefits of fasting further, it should be noted that this is just one tool in a toolbox of resources outlined in this book. It is provided in order for you to evaluate whether it fits into your own personal makeup. It doesn't have to be incorporated into your lifestyle, and it can be advisable to seek guidance from physicians if you are within certain demographics. But make no mistake—fasting is a powerful, valuable, yet too rarely used approach to health.

Fat Burning

One of the reasons that fasting is so worthwhile is that it can play a major role in shifting the body from a sugar burner to a fat burner. This is massively helpful, as any weight loss and health program should be centered on coaxing the body into a state of ketosis (i.e., fat burning). Achieving ketosis will help you get fitter, leaner, healthier, and feel great, so it's fantastic news that intermittent fasting can be a central part of this process.

But I know what you're thinking. Pretty much exactly the same things that I thought when I first heard about fasting. I can't do without food, it's not healthy to go for long periods without eating, this will just slow down my metabolism . . . okay, I hear you! We're going to explain and dispel all of these myths as we go along. Be reassured before we start that intermittent fasting actually achieves the opposite effects to those you have probably heard from the mainstream media and drug-pushing companies!

Fasting Myths

- Skipping meals will slow down your metabolism.
- Fasting puts your body in starvation mode.
- Fasting causes muscle loss.
- You will gain the weight back after eating.
- You will have lower energy without food.

First, fasting doesn't require some phenomenal feat of endurance. The best way to begin with intermittent fasting is to aim for a shortened eating schedule. Initially, this can be achieved by simply pushing back the time that you first eat by one hour or even 30 minutes. Similarly, you can stop eating one hour or 30 minutes earlier than usual at the end of the day. Then repeat this process on a regular basis, until you're eating all of your meals between the hours of 11 a.m. and 7 p.m.

Nothing New

It is worth remembering at this point that fasting is actually nothing new at all. We all go large blocks of time without eating every single day during an activity that you may have heard referred to as sleeping! Furthermore, it is notable that the Muslim community fasts quite extensively during Ramadan, and they ramp up the process further still by avoiding liquids as well. While this is not necessarily recommended from an ideal health perspective, we can also note that this has no disastrous impact on the well-being of that community.

Indeed, human beings have been fasting for thousands of years. In our high-calorie, carb-obsessed, snack-intensive culture it may seem unnatural, but eating every couple of hours is, in fact, an entirely new phenomenon from an evolutionary perspective. You only need to go back one generation in order to experience a time when children were rarely allowed to snack at all. I certainly wasn't permitted to do so when I was growing up!

We have since been trained, mostly by a combination of television and corporations, that snacking regularly is normal, and indeed we need to be cramming food into our mouths virtually every waking moment; otherwise, we will wither and die! Not only is this complete and utter nonsense, but it also has a hugely detrimental impact on our collective human health.

It is no coincidence that virtually every Western nation is experiencing a massive obesity and diabetes epidemic. The simple reason is that we don't eat healthy food and we don't consume it in a healthy way. A pretty bad combination! The onslaught of convenience food and marketing in the last 20 years has convinced us to snack on high-sugar, high-carb food, and this approach is often even advocated by physicians.

Certainly, the level of carbohydrates recommended by government bodies tends to be far higher than is actually necessary. As most doctors are provided with extremely limited nutritional education, they usually acquiesce with existing studies, which are all too often funded by the food industry. The system works!

Anyway, back to fasting . . .

Metabolism Myth

One of the most commonly promulgated myths regarding fasting is that we need to eat regularly in order to keep our metabolism ticking. You constantly need to put another log on the fire in order to keep it burning, right? While this is a convincing metaphor, the reality is that it certainly doesn't work in practice.

No doubt we've all been told on several occasions that if you skip a meal, your body will start virtually eating itself and your metabolism will slow to the pace of a slug. See a free video at www.yourhealthisnonnegotiable.com/freevideos where I explain how your metabolism works. Yet we now eat more often than at any time in human history, and we are demonstrably more out of shape, obese, unhealthy (and arguably unhappy) than ever before. Clearly, our current approach to food and nutrition isn't working.

So how do we really need to eat?

Supportive Studies

Well, the first thing to note is that it is extremely difficult to locate any studies that actively support regular eating. When you do find them—surprise, surprise!—they are all commissioned by companies such as ABC Big Business Food Co. I wonder what vested interest ABC Big Business Food Co might have in your snacking and eating on a regular basis . . .

I have found research to support the health benefits, and particularly fat-burning capabilities, of intermittent fasting. Engaging in intermittent fasting enables the body to reduce triglycerides[1] and decreased blood pressure,[2] while markers for inflammation are also significantly reduced.[3]

This latter point is important, as it leads to water loss, with inflamed tissue holding on to water and disrupting hormonal processes. Fasting is, therefore, a brilliant way to balance the hormone levels in your body, which is really the foundation for any health program.

Intermittent fasting can also deliver a reduction in oxidative stress. This fancy term can really be summarized as the rusting of the body, as it effectively represents aging at the cellular level. With more research being released by academics on an almost monthly basis, the support for the health benefits of fasting is growing ever stronger.

The Nobel Prize Winner

One particular esteemed example of this is the work of Professor Yoshinori Ohsumi. This Nobel Prize winner is an expert on the process of autophagy. This obscure word derived from the Greek for "self" and *phagein*, "to eat," refers to the anatomical process of the regulated and destructive mechanism of cells that disassembles unnecessary or dysfunctional components. To simplify that somewhat, it is a critical part of cell regeneration, which is a vital component of overall health.

Professor Ohsumi discovered that fasting greatly aids this process of autophagy. Nutrient deprivation is the key activator of autophagy,[4] due to the fact that insulin and glucagon have an inverse relationship. If insulin goes up, glucagon goes down. And as we eat, insulin goes up, and thus glucagon must go down. In fact, this process is disturbed in those suffering from type 2 diabetes.[5]

So when we fast, insulin levels go down and glucagon goes up. This increase in glucagon stimulates the process of autophagy. In fact, fasting provides the greatest known boost to autophagy.

Research has demonstrated that autophagy can even be achieved by supportive fasting (i.e., eating a controlled diet without undergoing the fasting process). This has been corroborated by research in both Japan and America, underlining the power of the full intermittent fasting procedure.

Weight Loss Is Not The Point

So fasting can be used for weight loss reasons, but it also offers a great deal more than merely weight benefits. The process can be used to increase cellular turnover,[6] which means that the body heals itself faster, making you feel better. This is one of the fundamental building blocks of human health, and as mentioned in the introduction, this book really provides a template for cellular health. What is going on inside you internally will ultimately dictate your external appearance and functioning, so although we often discount these processes, they are absolutely of critical importance.

Improved cellular turnover results in better nails, better hair, better skin, better vitality . . . essentially just a better you . . . period! It is undoubtedly one of the most compelling reasons to engage in intermittent fasting. But there are others as well.

As touched upon previously, fasting enables your metabolism to shift into fat-burning mode.[7] This transition into ketosis will help improve your metabolic flexibility, making it easier to stay in nutritional ketosis and remain in fat-burning mode longer. If one of your goals is to lose weight . . . trust me, this is great news!

Understandable Skepticism

Let me assure you that I have tested my own skepticism. It is not enough for me to see scientific surveys and the outcome of other people's experiences with intermittent fasting . . . I need to see it for myself!

So I experimented with fasting to see how this concept would fit with my lifestyle. As a rule, I can say that I normally practice a 14–20 hour fast daily and have fasted for up to four days in my experiment. Fasting is hard at first, but being fat-adapted before working at the fasting concept is a big advantage. People who practice the keto diet first can then slip into the fasting practice effortlessly because their bodies are not "jonesing" for sugar. Once your body is in a fat-adapted state, your body operates in a completely different state by living off sugar energy.

Your body was designed to use fat for fuel. It's the reserve of our system when food is not available during droughts and long winters. Fat can help insulate our bodies to help us stay warm and energized in order to survive the tough conditions that you witness wildlife living in today.

So if you feel any skepticism about the process of fasting, by all means, test out your own anatomy and see how it responds. I am in no way suggesting that everyone will respond in exactly the same way, and it is critical to understand your own body. But while the results of intermittent fasting may not be uniform across all people, you will see that they are rather similar in the vast majority of cases.

Appetite Control

There are many other benefits of intermittent fasting as well. One of the most attractive, particularly to those looking to lose weight, is that the process helps with appetite control by regulating the hunger hormones ghrelin and leptin. Before engaging in fasting, many people are understandably scared that they will experience unbearable hunger, yet intermittent fasting actually helps you to control hunger.[8]

Another benefit of intermittent fasting is that it will lower your blood glucose levels.[9] It has also been shown to boost neurogenesis and neuronal plasticity by offering protection against neurotoxins.[10] More is being learned about this and the benefits of intermittent fasting on our anatomical makeup, but there is clear evidence that this technique helps fight disease while keeping our bodies younger for a longer period.

Rebooted Immune System

There is also scientific evidence that fasting can improve your immune system. The Italian American biogerontologist and cell biologist Dr. Valter Longo has conducted extensive research on the role of fasting and nutrient response genes on cellular protection, aging, and diseases.[11] He found that engaging in a program of fasting can regenerate the immune system in as little as two days.[12] Within four days, it will help the body begin to fight off infection.

So in 72 hours, intermittent fasting will effectively provide you with a replenished immune system. The exciting thing about this is that this has also been demonstrated in those immune systems that have been heavily damaged by chemotherapy.[13] Research indicates that fasting can diminish the growth of tumors,[14] while studies on both mice and humans indicate that the process lowers white blood cell count.[15]

Intermittent fasting can also assist with the problem of a leaky gut.[16] We dive deeper into what leaky gut is in our gut health chapter, but this is all to say that fasting can help with the absorption of nutrients. What fasting essentially achieves is the creation of a clean-slate condition for the gut, meaning that you can manage your digestive system much more effectively.

Understand Your Own Body

Intermittent fasting may not necessarily be right for everyone. It is vital to understand your own body and treat it in the appropriate fashion that suits you. Equally, it should be stated that most people who embark on a fasting journey experience tremendous success.

As you experiment, note that intermittent fasting should be phased in gradually due to its impact on hormonal levels. The week prior to fasting you can begin by reducing your carb intake, hydrating the body as much as possible, and eating lots of salads and nourishing soups. As you come out of a fast, do not dive for the cupboard, as you might suffer from a crazy insulin crash. Also, have all your meals prepared well in advance so that you can ease into eating again without feeling famished.

With this in mind, when engaging in a program of intermittent fasting, you should avoid anything that will tend to kick your body out of the state of ketosis. While there isn't a perfect plan to follow here, as it differs from person to person, it can be said with some confidence that higher carbohydrate, protein, and calorie intake will tend to result in the body beginning to burn glucose rather than fat. Over time, it will be possible for you to recognize that your body is in fat-burning mode, so it really is a case of trial and error and getting to know one's own physique. Another important note is that you want to be mindful of the consumption of protein as well. Protein in large amounts can be converted into glucose in a process called gluconeogenesis. This is the process that leads to the generation of glucose from a variety of sources such as pyruvate, lactate, glycerol, and certain amino acids.

Let's take some time now to debunk and address some of the other myths you've heard about fasting.

Myth 1: Health Hazards

As I mentioned earlier, it is often strongly stated that any form of fasting can be dangerous and hazardous to your health. The reality is that it is actually completely safe and beneficial, but it is important to note some risks as well.

Intermittent fasting experts advise that breastfeeding mothers, those who suffer from eating disorders, diabetics, children, those with less than 5 percent body fat to lose, and those with metabolic disorders should avoid intermittent fasting. For most people, there is no risk whatsoever as long as they consume their vitamins, minerals, and water daily.

Myth 2: Weight Loss And Fasting

Does intermittent fasting help with weight loss? Yes, you will lose weight. But this shouldn't be seen as the overarching purpose of intermittent fasting, let alone the sole motivation. Fasting is one way to achieve weight loss over time with consistent safe practice, but it should be accompanied by several other tools. Fasting should instead be seen as a way of improving your overall anatomy, with increased gut permeability, metabolic function, and reduced body fat being some key benefits.

Fasting is obviously helpful in the ongoing battle to achieve weight loss, but should not be viewed as a silver bullet. Also, it is important to note that some weight that you lose from intermittent fasting will come back. This is water weight, and it is supposed to return.

The important thing is that if you combine intermittent fasting with a diet low in carbohydrates, you will burn through your glucose stores rather rapidly. Indeed, intermittent fasting can result in beginning the process of ketosis in as little as 24 hours. This then makes it easier to enter nutritional ketosis and stay in fat-burning mode. This will definitely assist with your weight loss goals, but more importantly, it will be hugely beneficial for your overall health and cellular functioning.

Remember, we are not restricting calories here. During your feeding windows, you should be fueling the body with the adequate calories based on your metabolic rate, and it should be noted that sneaking in snacks will certainly break your fast. Don't be fooled into thinking that just a "small bite won't hurt." This detracts from the true benefits of a fast. During a true fast, you would consume only water. Some people drink teas and bone broths to get by. Tip: don't add any artificial or natural sweeteners to your waters and teas, as this will mess with your messaging reward centers and very possibly ignite some hunger growls of ghrelin.

Myth 3: You Will Regain The Weight

One of the most commonly advanced myths related to intermittent fasting is that you will regain any weight lost almost immediately. As mentioned previously, you can expect your water weight to return, and this is an entirely healthy process. There is absolutely no reason whatsoever why your body fat should return! It cannot just magically come back out of thin air!

You can expect to lose half a pound of body fat on a daily basis while fasting, as the process forces the body to access your fat stores. While intermittent fasting can require some adaptation, it also improves your biochemical systems and prompts mitochondrial regeneration.[17] The reason that fasting works so well is that it gets your body functioning better internally so you reap the rewards with external benefits.

Myth 4: Your Muscles Will Dissipate During Fasting

This one is a complete myth, as fasting actually results in an increase in human growth hormone (HGH) production.[18] In fact, this can be as much as 500 percent compared to non-fasting nutritional programs. Fasting, in fact, aids the body in muscle development, as it forces the pituitary gland to secrete HGH.

This is of critical importance, as HGH promotes the usage of fat for energy, effectively creating a leaner physique while diminishing inflammation. It even decreases hunger levels and increases bone density,[19] so the notion that fasting will destroy your muscularity is absolute nonsense!

SUMMARY

In conclusion, we have seen that fasting can have numerous positive impacts on the body, as well as being a worthwhile tool in achieving any weight loss goals that you might have. But don't run off to start fasting just yet! Before you engage in a program of intermittent fasting, it is important to consider the four following factors:

1. Are you doing this for the right reasons? Intermittent fasting should be viewed as part of an overall program to improve the cellular makeup of your body, not as an easy way to lose weight. If you are simply fasting alone, with no other support or backup strategies, purely to

achieve weight loss, then you should probably think again about your approach.

2. Instead, intermittent fasting should be undertaken in order to transform your body into an effective fat burner. This typically happens at around the 20–30-hour mark, although it can vary from person to person. This should be a key motivation in any intermittent fasting program, as it is really the underlying aim of the process.

3. Another major benefit of intermittent fasting is to improve the immune system. This should be considered a critical aspect of any fasting program, as it is going to get your body working as it should. Our immune systems should be powerful and effective; unfortunately, we bombard them with so much chemical crap that this isn't always the case. Fasting effectively provides a reset switch for your anatomy.

4. Alongside the immune system, intermittent fasting also has a massively positive impact on gut health, assisting with problems such as leaky gut and ensuring that the digestive system functions far more effectively.

These are the four major reasons to engage in a program of intermittent fasting. So I really hope that you will overcome your initial skepticism and resistance to this concept and give it a go. It is also important to pay close attention to the guidance and advice presented in this chapter, especially for those in high-risk groups. Everyone's bodies are different, and they shouldn't be treated in the uniform fashion that is common in mainstream advice.

But I really believe that fasting is a powerful tool, one that is wrongly demonized, and a process that can be hugely beneficial for your body as a whole. However, it is even more effective when used in conjunction with the exciting approach that I'm going to outline in the rest of the book. So let's crack on and dive into them!

Challenger Story

Tamara has her own very personal story to share. It is inspiring because it demonstrates that no matter how challenging your circumstances may be, our six-week program can get you back on track and, ultimately, to where you want to be.

When we first met Tamara, she was struggling with polycystic ovary syndrome (PCOS) and hypothyroidism, while she had also recently been informed of the early onset of menopause. This trifecta, triple-whammy, of hormonal conditions was seriously debilitating for her, and she was struggling with her weight and health.

In fact, Tamara's doctor had recommended hormone treatment in tablet form before she was introduced to our program. I am so glad that she was, as we've been able to play a major role in turning her life around completely.

One of the inspiring things for Tamara is that she was initially reluctant to join a group class. She felt that she would have to go at her own pace and wasn't keen on being around what she perceived to be more physically competent people. But she was actually inspired by the community we have built. In her own words: ". . . fell in love with the way that the people I came into contact with help each other out."

The other big positive for Tamara has been the overhaul of her diet. She thought she already had a pretty good handle on the food she was eating. She considered herself reasonably healthy. But her habits have been transformed since then.

Tamara found that fasting played a particularly prominent role in her health transformation. Allowing the body to rest from digestion helped to rapidly and radically reduce her internal inflammation. Changing her diet reduced her body fat and ensured that she didn't have to rely on medication to control her PCOS.

The supportive community that we have built, which is a huge source of pride for me, has also played a massive role in Tamara's transformation. She has made friends for life, and notes that the common goals shared by the people involved, along with the camaraderie, ensure that you achieve excellent results.

Tamara has set herself on a path to health redemption, along with countless other people who have benefited from this unique program of physical transformation.

Chapter Three

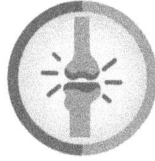

INFLAMMATION
THE GOAL THIS WEEK (WEEK TWO):
TO REDUCE INFLAMMATION

1. Discover the foods that are causing inflammation in your body.

2. Further increase fasting windows.

IN THE PREVIOUS CHAPTER OF THIS BOOK, WE LOOKED AT THE VALUE OF FASTING. There was a reason that we introduced this first, as it paves the way for addressing inflammation in the body. This is part of a three-step process, which will be completed by addressing the health of your gut in the next chapter.

It is invaluable to begin by fasting, as this assists the body in the healing process from the inflammation that it will no doubt have accrued. Once you have addressed all three prongs of this approach, you can expect the way you feel to have improved considerably. Yay for you!

But for now, let's stick to the job at hand and deal with the critical topic of inflammation.

Your Steps To Success

Step 1: Select and prepare in advance your chosen recipes for the week.

Step 2: Limit the food choices this week. It's time to become a detective. The more variety you have in the foods you are consuming, the harder it is to identify the ones causing inflammation.

Step 3: Take before-and-after pictures of your face on Sunday and then the following Sunday. Look for signs of inflammation.

Tips

1. Remove dairy this week and preferably for the rest of the program. Dairy is well known for causing inflammation.

2. Remove anything with gluten in the ingredients, but ALWAYS check the labels. Just because a label says gluten-free on it does not mean that the other ingredients included are healthy. You can watch the free video on food labels at www.yourhealthisnonnegotiable.com/freevideos.

3. We do want to reduce and minimize fruits as we progress through the program for their sugar content,

but in this case, we also want to be very mindful of any pesticides.

4. Stick to non-starchy carbs (green salads) to help reduce stored fat and water retention.

5. Hydration is, of course, very important. Keep the body well hydrated to help flush away toxins, free radicals, and to keep the body well lubricated, so that it may function at its peak performance. Aim to consume 500 ml four to five times a day.

6. Keep the body in motion. Try to build muscle. The stronger your muscles are around your joints, the less pain you may experience if you suffer from an "-itis."

7. Focus on reducing stress, and focus heavily on getting seven to eight hours of sleep a night as much as possible in order to help the body heal and repair.

BE MINDFUL OF THE FOLLOWING INFLAMMATORY SYMPTOMS:

- How often do you feel gassy and bloated?

- How often do you suffer from flatulence?

- How often do you have a stuffy nose?

- How often do you feel excess mucus production in your head and throat?

- Are you noticing swelling around your joints?

- Are you suffering from headaches?

- Do you have sore hands or feet?

- Are you experiencing muscle soreness or joint pain?

- Are you suffering from mood swings or depression?

- Do you have itchy skin or skin rashes?

- Are you having stomach pains? If so, you may suffer from IBS, ulcerative colitis, or Crohn's disease.

THE SCIENCE

What Is Inflammation?

It is important to note that inflammation is a perfectly natural process. It is intended to protect the body against viruses and wounds and is essentially part of the body's ability to heal itself. If you look in a dictionary under "inflammation," it will be defined as the "pathophysiology underlying most chronic diseases." *Pathophysiology* is a fancy medical term that simply means the anatomical processes associated with disease or injury.

While inflammation is perfectly natural, and sometimes healthy, the extent to which people in the West are now suffering from internal inflammation certainly is not. The diet we are consuming in this modern society is leading to extremely undesirable levels of inflammation, and many people are suffering from this debilitating condition without even realizing it.

Luckily, it is not difficult to counter inflammation via anti-inflammatory foods. The human body is a great healer, and the level of inflammation within our anatomies can actually be reduced pretty rapidly. While you may not realize that you are exhibiting some symptoms of inflammation, these too can be reduced, and eventually eliminated, simply by addressing the underlying cause.

Two Types of Inflammation

Inflammation basically comes down to two separate types: acute and chronic. Needless to say, chronic inflammation is more serious, potentially lasting for years. Chronic inflammation is caused by pathogens that the body cannot break down, including some types of virus, foreign bodies that remain in the system, or overactive immune responses.

But that doesn't mean that the consequences of acute inflammation are to be ignored. Acute inflammation will eventually develop into chronic inflammation if it is not addressed. The cause of acute inflammation is harmful bacteria or tissue injuries (we'll look into the root cause of inflammation imminently). The onset of acute inflammation is rapid, and although it often only lasts a few days, the potential seriousness of this issue should not be underestimated.

What Causes Inflammation?

The reason that our bodies so often create inflammation in contemporary society is that foreign particles are entering them that simply aren't supposed to be present. This naturally causes disruption. Unfortunately, much of this destruction comes from our diets; it is not a temporary scenario for many people.

Environmental toxins can also be a contributing factor, but the fact is that most body discomfort comes directly from the food that we put into our bodies. I mean, we've all heard the expression "You are what you eat"—right? Well, there is a reason that this idiom came into being: it is a particularly illustrative way of emphasizing the importance of carefully monitoring the foods you consume.

Unfortunately, in our hectic modern culture, we too rarely pay attention to this critical aspect of human health. As mentioned in the previous chapter, we are incentivized by some extremely powerful and wealthy interests to engage in behavior that is essentially damaging to our health.

Indeed, the statistics on inflammation are quite sobering. The level of inflammation that is now common in society is underlined by the fact that America spends approximately $3.5 trillion annually on health care.[1] (Of course, this shouldn't ever be referred to as "health care," as it doesn't address underlying health issues! It should be called sick care! But I digress ...)

Despite spending this vast amount of money on treating illness, the United States remains one of the unhealthiest nations in the Western world. It ranks rock bottom among industrialized countries in all-around health, suffering from more degenerative diseases than any other country on the planet. In America, 50 percent of people will die of heart attacks and strokes[2] and 33 percent will contract cancer,[3] while one in eight women will contract breast cancer.[4]

Cellular Level

One of the important contextual issues to understand with inflammation is that all problems of this nature begin at the cellular level and with the body's internal functioning. While our DNA has the ability to mutate over thousands of years, it is no match for the rapidly evolving food environment that has emerged in the last few decades. This industrialized food production system has certainly produced a large quantity of food, but it can also be held primarily responsible for our declining health.

This means that before you begin any process of addressing inflammation, it is always worthwhile to take a food sensitivity and allergy test. This will address whether you have any underlying problems and can play a critical role in your future diet and well-being.

Toxic Food Environment

Dr. Kelly Brownell, dean of the Sanford School of Public Policy at Duke University, and Robert L. Flowers, professor of public policy, professor of psychology and neuroscience, and director of the World Food Policy Center, describe the contemporary climate as a "toxic food environment," and assert that we live in an environment that almost "100 percent guarantees that we become sick."[5] I certainly agree with this verdict, but the good news is that we can fight back against this toxic culture. Hurray! Finally some good news!

The best way to address internal inflammation, as I mentioned earlier, is with a food-based approach. While there are other anti-inflammatory lifestyle elements available, the problem is almost without exception a fundamental issue of diet, and this can be addressed very rapidly by simply eating healthier foods.

As you are no doubt learning by now—if you didn't know already!—everyone's body is different. There is no uniform way of treating the human anatomy; there is always some variation from one person's body to another. All of our DNA codes are different; all of our lineages are different. We are all exposed to different environmental elements throughout our lives, and there are a variety of other factors which ensure that our response to food can be quite significantly different.

Your body is unique, and this should be seen as a wonderful thing! Pat yourself on the back! But it does mean that there is no truly one-size-fits-all solution! No matter how much people with a vested interest may claim otherwise, there really isn't!

What Are the Physical Effects of Inflammation?

If you think about this in terms of an analogy, inflammation is similar to our skin swelling when it is wounded. Tolerating this for a short period would not be considered too alarming, but if our skin were to be permanently swollen, then this would become rather worrisome and obviously indicate an underlying problem. So you can assume immediately that our insides are not meant to be permanently inflamed either and that getting our body back to a state of natural health involves eliminating this undesirable condition.

When considering inflammation, it is important to understand the long-term consequences of this condition. We are not talking about some minor inconvenience here! This is serious stuff, so listen carefully!

Diseases such as diabetes, heart disease, and cancer, along with a wide variety of autoimmune conditions, can be considered evidence that the body is desperately fighting inflammation.[6] Furthermore, as most of these conditions can be considered degenerative, it also suggests that in most cases the anatomical systems have been fighting inflammation for quite some time. Considering that all forms of inflammation are intended to be a temporary defense mechanism, this is not a healthy state of affairs.

What Are the Hazardous Effects of Inflammation?

Inflammation can have a wide range of knock-on effects on the body and its functioning, many of which can be extremely negative. It probably won't come as a huge surprise to learn that inflammation damages the gut. This can eventually trigger inflammatory bowel disease, which includes ulcerative colitis and Crohn's disease. Symptoms of this include bloating, diarrhea, cramps, and ulcers.

Joint problems and rheumatoid arthritis can also result from inflammation, while the condition has also been linked with heart disease. A 2012 study in *The Lancet* noted that when chronic inflammation occurs due to problems with the arteries heart attacks can follow. Even those who experience chronic inflammation due to an autoimmune disorder have a higher risk of heart disease.

Cancer has also been linked with chronic inflammation, particularly in a 2014 Harvard University study. Researchers from the esteemed university discovered that obese teenagers with high levels of inflammation had a 63 percent increased risk of developing colorectal cancer during adulthood.

Inflammation is also bad for your lungs, causing fluid accumulation and narrowing of the airways, making it harder to breathe. Inflammation can also damage your gums, make weight loss more difficult, promote increased bone loss, cause skin problems such as psoriasis, and even lead to mental health conditions such as depression. Overall, inflammation is definitely something to avoid.

How Exercise Causes Inflammation, but in a Good Way

The long-term impact on our physiology is entirely grim. Bodies become inflamed in order to help protect underlying systems, but when our digestive system is being bombarded with inflammatory food, this is extremely difficult to deal with. But, conversely, short-term inflammation can be good for the body—think exercise, for example.

Indeed, some inflammation is required if a workout is to achieve anything meaningful. Hypertrophy, increased stamina, increased strength, and improved work capacity all require some degree of inflammation in order to occur. Your body essentially strengthens itself via the inflammatory response to stress and by strengthening and rebuilding its tissues in order to cope with future demands.

Any advanced training session is essentially an acute stressor that provokes an inflammatory response from the body. But, crucially, this effect is fleeting and non-permanent, resulting in a powerful short-term response.

What Foods and Products Cause Inflammation in the Body?

Long-term inflammation, though, is often caused by poor diet. Yet many of us don't even realize that we're eating unhealthy food, let alone that it's causing inflammation. Unfortunately, we have been led up the garden path with regard to nutrition, and millions, if not billions, of people, are now consuming toxic foods without even knowing it. Thus, it's hardly surprising that their insides are inflamed.

Luckily, we do know what causes inflammation and what to avoid, so here is my guide to the key food groups and types to avoid during this six-week program (and to eliminate, or at the very least reduce, on a permanent basis).

Dairy

The first food group that you should particularly beware of is lactose and dairy, and there are several reasons for this. First, dairy is one of the food groups that will most likely cause people to experience an allergic reaction. It can be quite reasonably argued that there is absolutely no need to consume milk in the first place; indeed, no other mammal consumes the milk of other animals, let alone well into adulthood! Again, there is now a massive industry that has been built up around the production of dairy products, meaning that they have become part of our overall diets. But there are other compelling reasons to avoid, or at least minimize, dairy as well.

As mentioned previously, you have the problems associated with the feeding of dairy cattle, meaning there is always a possibility that you are effectively ingesting unknown chemicals. Different breeds of cow also produce different enzymes, with certain dairy products emanating from certain cows resulting in various dietary problems. Dairy products are actually endemically associated with causing inflammation, even before you consider the pesticides, chemicals, growth hormones, and other unnatural aspects of modern dairy farming.

So you may very well have been told that milk is healthy and a vital source of calcium, but you should certainly think twice before putting it into your body, at least in large quantities.

Sugar

Carbohydrates are, of course, massively linked with sugar, and it is this sweet substance that is the fourth group of which we should particularly be aware when addressing inflammation. Sugar is arguably the most important of all the groups that cause inflammation, simply because there are phenomenal amounts of the substance contained within contemporary food.

This has probably been the biggest revolution in the way that we eat, as refined and processed sugar was virtually nonexistent just 100 years ago. A commonly cited statistic is that the average American consumed only 5 percent of the sugar that is consumed today at that time.[7] Clearly, the body cannot evolve rapidly enough over a 100-year period in order to deal with a 20-fold increase in sugar consumption.

We are literally feeding the malaise of our bodies with this excessive sugar consumption, and addressing this should be considered absolutely critical in solving inflammation problems. In the previous chapter we talked about fasting, and you will notice that once you engage in a fast that you will lose several pounds immediately. This is literally because our bodies store up inflammation in the form of sugars, and this then dissipates rapidly when we deny our anatomy this addictive (yet admittedly delicious!) substance.

This is one of the big problems with sugar—it tastes good! Our bodies crave it because they know they're getting a supercharged burst of energy from it, and throughout most of human history, food was scarce. You couldn't just pop down to KFC and pick up a 5,000-calorie Bargain Bucket! Our bodies are not evolved enough to cope with the contemporary food environment, and they will fool us into eating poorly if we allow this to happen.

While there is more awareness now of the amount of added sugar in supermarket products, we are still consuming far too much. Educating yourself about the amount of added sugar in commonly consumed products should be considered absolutely essential. Cakes and desserts should be consumed rarely, and soda should never be consumed at all. Okay, if you're offered a choice between poison and soda, then it might be okay to pick soda, but you should probably just pass on both! Diet soda is not a healthy alternative! Aspartame, high-fructose corn syrup—to be frank, they are worse than the regular products.

Trans Fats

Trans fats are another byproduct of our contemporary food system and cooking processes, and these can cause massive inflammation in the human anatomy. These substances are new to our bodies and indeed this world, as they are derived from the process of deep-frying with cheap vegetable oils.[8]

While we can eliminate trans fats in our homes, we may also encounter difficulties with these substances in restaurants. Many commercial eateries will ramp up your trans-fat levels by deep-frying their food. You may wish to avoid restaurants completely, or at least be very selective about where you eat out. There is a tendency to cook with bad oils in restaurants, and once you experience the light and airy feeling that you will achieve from this program, you may decide against eating out altogether. Maybe grab a coffee instead of assaulting your body with sugar and trans fats.

Gluten

Avoiding gluten is something that many people are considering nowadays, with the tennis player Novak Djokovic being one example. Inflammation is common in an estimated three million adults and children in the United States who suffer from celiac disease, and millions more are also believed to be sensitive to gluten. This is a massive problem area and one that you should certainly address if you're aiming to eliminate inflammation.

Gluten is not fully digested by the body, and this can cause the immune system to view it as a foreign intruder and attack it. This then has the unfortunate consequence of causing inflammation in the intestine, and often other organs and tissues as well. Those suffering from celiac disease will suffer particularly badly, as gluten will trigger a powerful autoimmune response that damages the small intestine and negatively impacts its ability to absorb nutrients.

Ultimately, the inflammation caused by gluten can lead to weight loss, anemia, osteoporosis, infertility and miscarriage, skin rashes, headache, depression, fibromyalgia, and joint pain. This is why gluten is one of the most important substances to avoid if you want to beat inflammation.

Refined Carbohydrates

The third food group that can particularly cause inflammation is refined carbohydrates. This refers to sugars and starches that don't exist in nature. They do come from natural whole foods, but they have been altered in some way by processing, in order to "refine" them. Truly whole grains are intact kernels complete with their outer bran coating, as found in nature. Once the grain is broken into pieces by any kind of processing, it can be considered refined to some extent.

Refined carbohydrates are rapidly absorbed into the bloodstream, causing risky spikes in blood sugar and insulin levels.[9] They are mostly associated with products such as white bread and pasta, crackers, cakes, cookies, and bagels, but there are many other sources of refined carbs as well. An exhaustive list of refined carbohydrate products can be found online, and it is certainly advisable to avoid these or have them as an occasional treat.

GMO

Additionally, most processed foods contain corn, wheat, and soy, and thus they should be avoided. These food products are also often GMO (genetically modified organisms, meaning that they contain material that has been essentially created by science rather than grown by nature), which is another bone of contention. It can be reasonably stated that the scientific jury is still out on the long-term health impacts of genetically modified foods, but considering what we know about our bodies and DNA, it does seem that they are more likely to cause difficulties such as inflammation.

Regardless of this, what can be said with cast-iron certainty is that foods grown with genetically modified ingredients are far more likely to be exposed to chemicals. Such pesticides are a massive problem, as they contribute to killing good bacteria, which effectively wrecks our immune system. It has been documented that those foods grown with GMO will have a 95 percent chance of being treated with pesticides,[10] which in my book means that you should absolutely avoid them.

Changing the molecular structure that we have been consuming in our diets for thousands of years will undoubtedly cause problems in the body. Food that has been tampered with by human beings generally has negative impacts, and sadly we are dealing with a culture in which there is a huge amount of chemicalized food. And this is getting worse, not better, decade by decade.

Alcohol

You perhaps shouldn't be surprised to see this on the list, as you can literally fatally poison yourself with alcohol! It should therefore be rather obvious that alcohol is damaging to our insides. While drinking in moderation is still acceptable, depending on your susceptibility, it is quite easy for alcohol to enable bacteria to pass through the intestinal lining. This leads to irritation and inflammation, meaning that you should carefully monitor your alcohol consumption.

Corn and Soy

Our bodies are not necessarily designed to absorb corn and soybeans. This means that any consumption of these common products should be undertaken with care.

In particular, cattle are now frequently fed corn and soy,[11] as American farmers now create a surplus of this produce due to subsidization—another fantastic example of the system working wonderfully well! It is fairly common knowledge that a cow's stomach is a particularly intricate mechanism, intended to be fed with grass. This means that some supermarket products will now boast that they come direct from grass-fed cows as if this is some sort of achievement! Of course, all cows should be fed on grass, all the time!

By feeding cattle with corn and soybeans, we are causing inflammation within their anatomies and then often eating the muscles of their inflamed bodies. I'm sure that you have already deduced that this is not exactly good news for our health.

What Foods Help to Reduce Inflammation?

However, not only can you do something about this, but I'd also like to strike a note of optimism here. Resistance and opposition to the toxic food environment are growing as awareness and information about the food production system spread more freely. As the way we eat and produce food has evolved extremely rapidly, so has awareness of the industrialized system and processes involved.

If you think back to around 20 years ago, there would have been massive opposition, and possibly even ridicule, aimed at any form of food activism. A group of Greenpeace activists who fought the McDonald's corporation in Britain in the well-documented McLibel case were initially ridiculed by the media and personally attacked. Yet they became heroes after a lengthy court case, which caused considerable embarrassment to the fast-food chain.[12]

Today, there is simply far more awareness of the dangers of fast food and other unhealthy aspects of our food production system, and this does suggest that resistance and opposition are growing, though the food-producing corporations remain hugely powerful. Hopefully, this book can be part of an overall process of the turning of the tide against unhealthy and unnecessarily chemicalized and destructive food.

Here are some particular areas that I would like you to focus on when recalibrating your diet to avoid inflammation.

High Fiber

Any high-fiber foods are to be highly recommended. Cruciferous vegetables are particularly consistent with this, and there are other benefits to getting plenty of veggies. Cruciferous vegetables are vegetables of the family *Brassicaceae* and include arugula, bok choy, broccoli, brussels sprouts, cabbage, cauliflower, collard greens, kale, kohlrabi, maca, mizuna, mustard greens, radish, rutabaga, turnip, and watercress. Some of those names may seem highly exotic and unfamiliar, but trust me, they're all good!

Cruciferous vegetables also help regulate blood sugar levels and tend to promote weight loss,[13] while they have been shown to be a big cancer fighter as well. Cruciferous vegetables pack in plenty of antioxidants that can help neutralize cancer-causing free radicals and also contain compounds like glucosinolates and indole-3-carbinol, which have been shown to help fight off cancer.[14] A minimum of four to five servings per day of beets, carrots, cruciferous vegetables (broccoli, cabbage, cauliflower and kale), dark leafy greens (collard greens, kale, spinach), onions, peas, salad greens, sea vegetables, and squash is recommended.

Resveratrol and Curcumin

These two substances are probably not widely known. (In fact, the spellchecker has just underlined them both, so it's obviously never heard of them!) Resveratrol is actually produced by numerous plants as a response to injury and is thus great at assisting with inflammation. It is also found naturally in red wine, so it's a great excuse to get drunk! (That was a joke, by the way.)

Organic red wine in moderation can provide you with access to resveratrol, and this will not only help with inflammation but it also decreases the risk of heart disease. Scientists have found that the substance regenerates the body at the cellular level,[15] which, as we've discussed previously, is really the building block of all good health. If you're not keen on wine, then the substance can also be found in raw cocoa and dark berries, such as lingonberries, blueberries, mulberries, and bilberries.

Seasonal Food

As a brief aside: if possible, it is always beneficial to consume seasonal food. Supermarkets now seemingly offer every single type of food all year round and are extremely good at marketing things with colorful displays and packaging.

This has meant that where our ancestors would consume around 250 species in their diets, these would be seasonal and local,[16] and they regularly engaged in fasting cycles, the picture is very different today. Very few of us engage in fasting, and the typical supermarket consumer eats around 50 species during the average year. There has been a disastrous diminution in the diversity of food that we are consuming, and the level of indulgence associated with food is, frankly, completely out of control. It is always amusing to me that Christmas is seen as a time to stuff yourself with rich food, as I always wonder how this makes it different from any of the other days of the year!

In short, life was completely and utterly different from today for thousands and thousands of years. In many ways, and contrary to the messages we tend to receive from mainstream sources, the huge changes in our diet are most dramatic. Luckily, it is not difficult to retrain our bodies into a healthy lifestyle, but it is necessary to see beyond what we know and generally experience on a daily basis in order to achieve this.

Healthy Fats and Oils

Healthy fats and oils should be considered an essential part of an anti-inflammation program. Cheap vegetable oils that are sold in supermarkets are extremely unhealthy, resulting in trans fats when heated to high temperatures. These are absolutely to be avoided, and other options such as hemp oil, avocado oil, grapeseed oil, and many other healthier oils should be purchased instead. All of this may seem a culture shock at first, but you will quickly find that food tastes better when cooked in these substances.

Omega-3 Fatty Acids

Omega-3 fatty acids have long been recognized as superfood substances, conferring many health benefits on those who consume them. Omega-3s have been shown to lower blood pressure, while they also possess positive benefits for our hearts. The substances can also have a beneficial impact on our appearance, as they tend to improve our skin, hair, and nails. There are hundreds of promising trials that are charting the positive effects of omega-3s on Alzheimer's, ADHD, depression, and children's learning and behavior.[17]

Research also indicates that omega-3 fatty acids help reduce inflammation[18] and have a positive impact on autoimmune diseases. Omega-3s can be acquired through oily fish such as salmon, and there is a wide range of supplements also available. Other sources of omega-3s include walnuts, canola oil, sardines, chia seeds, mackerel, and flaxseeds.

Protein

Protein is an essential part of reducing inflammation, but it is absolutely critical to acquire this substance from a healthy source. No growth hormones, no genetically modified ingredients, no unwanted chemicals. We should consume around four to eight ounces of protein on a daily basis, and this is perfectly possible regardless of whether we consume meat or not. Nonetheless, poultry, red meat, and fish are obviously good sources of protein, but other alternatives are seitan, tofu, lentils, chickpeas, beans, yeast, spelt, teff, hempseed, green peas, spirulina, amaranth, quinoa, oatmeal, wild rice, chia seeds, pretty much all nuts, broccoli, spinach, asparagus, artichokes, potatoes, sweet potatoes, and brussels sprouts. Be sure that if you are consuming proteins from animals, your sources have been verified to be local, clean, organic farms that are humanely raising the animals in a natural environment and feeding them with foods they were designed to eat. I won't go into this tangent now, but trust me, it's extremely important to your health.

Organic Drinks

Organic drinks such as wine, juices, and teas can also play a major role in reducing inflammation. Organic ingredients will help you avoid unwanted and undesirable chemicals. It is always important to ensure that you are fully hydrated at all times as well, and selecting appropriate liquids is obviously extremely important in this regard. You should also pay heed to the amount of sugar that you are consuming through liquids.

Bone Broth

Bone broth has fantastic restorative properties for your gut, but also has an overall positive influence on your body as a whole. It supports a healthy immune system and also assists with leaky gut, a condition that we're going to get into in considerable detail in the next chapter.

This foodstuff is particularly beneficial for inflammation, as the collagen and gelatin substances contained in bone broth, along with the amino acids proline, glutamine, and arginine, can play a major role in sealing any opening that you may have developed in your intestine. This supports overall gut integrity, which will greatly help with the fight against inflammation.

Berries

Berries can also make a contribution to easing inflammation, whether you prefer blueberries, raspberries, strawberries, blackberries, or huckleberries. The antioxidant components of these berries, such as proanthocyanidins and ellagic acid, help your body fight inflammation and repair cell damage. Variety is also key here, as the amount and combination of the beneficial compounds differ from one berry to another.

Water

I've already made it clear how important hydration is in any healthy body. Our bodies are mainly comprised of water, and thus if you neglect to hydrate your body, then you can't possibly expect it to work properly. Sorry, it just won't!

Water is key to your overall inflammation strategy. And health professionals will all tell you without exception that keeping yourself hydrated is critical to many aspects of health. So make sure that you do it!

Beans and Legumes

Beans and lentils are also a valuable superfood in this area, while you should also consider consuming nuts and seeds, pulses, and hot peppers. It is quite easy to get a lot of good fiber into your body, making a massive difference to inflammation.

Healthy Herbs and Spices

Finally, in this section, healthy herbs and spices are also valuable inflammation fighters. These ingredients contain a liberal dose of antioxidants, minerals, and vitamins, which help you to maximize the nutrient content of your meals. Additionally, studies have shown that spices tend to have unique medicinal qualities. Researchers discovered that four spices—cloves, ginger, rosemary, and turmeric—were particularly effective at inducing an inflammatory response in white blood cells.

Another study published in the *Journal of Medicinal Foods* noted that spice and herb extracts can inhibit glycation and block the formation of advanced glycation end-products. This research suggested that cloves, cinnamon, Jamaican allspice, apple-pie spice mixture, oregano, pumpkin-pie spice mixture, marjoram, sage, thyme, and gourmet Italian spice are particularly potent anti-inflammatory herbs and spices.

Next, I want to provide you with a checklist of both anti-inflammatory foods and those foodstuffs that tend to cause problems in a lot of people's guts.

ANTI-INFLAMMATORY FOODS LIST

Non-starchy vegetables

Grass-fed, grass-finished beef

Berries

Extra-virgin olive oil

MCT oil

Avocados

Raw nuts and seeds

Bone broth

Ghee

Lemons and limes

Wild-caught salmon

Unrefined coconut oil

Herbs and spices

Whole eggs

POTENTIAL INTOLERANCES FOR SOME PEOPLE

Eggs

Kombucha

Caffeine

Chocolate

Beans

Vinegar

Dairy

Grains

Stevia

Citrus fruits

Coffee

Some nuts

Carbonated beverages

Guar or xanthan gums

Organic fermented soy

Nightshade vegetables

INFLAMMATORY FOODS LIST

Gluten

Alcohol

Grains

Dairy

Soy

Peanuts

Soda

Fast food

Fried foods

Artificial colors or dyes

Sugar and high-fructose corn syrup

Artificial sweeteners

Vegetable oils

Smoked, canned, or processed meat

Refined carbohydrates

Jams, jellies, syrups

Hydrogenated oils

"Fruit" beverages not containing 100 percent juice

Conventionally raised animal foods

The topic of inflammation could really justify an entire book in itself. Sadly, it is both a fundamental and hidden part of the human experience, particularly in North America. While suffering from internal inflammation is a common experience throughout the Western world, it is undoubtedly more prevalent in the United States in particular.

There is a very simple reason for this: food sold in the United States, and consequently the diet of American people, is worse than anywhere in the world—more chemicalized, more sugar-ridden, more processed, and unhealthier. That's why some of the most alarming statistics related to the United States are completely unique to the nation. The level of osteoporosis, autoimmune disease, heart ailments, and cancer in the US are now completely off the chart, and this can mostly be attributed to poor diet.

Indeed, it is common for people in countries such as Okinawa, China, and Indonesia to live far longer than Americans and ultimately pass away due to old age. This is the perfectly natural state for the body and human existence, particularly in an age where many dangerous diseases from the past have been completely eradicated. We are not dying now due to typhoid, for example; we are dying due to our own unhealthy lifestyles.

Luckily, our bodies are also extremely resistant and profoundly skilled at healing themselves, and the information in this chapter will help you get back on the right road to healing inflammation in your body. Phew!

Challenger Story

Sandra had hit rock bottom when we first came into contact with her. This is a common theme with lots of people that we work with, and it feels so good to be able to help them out of the rut that they've experienced.

Life was tough for Sandra when she found us. She had recently lost her job, and on top of that, her health had measurably declined. This is natural during a stressful time, but Sandra was literally in chronic pain when she first came to us.

Having encountered massive difficulties in her professional life, with a job that didn't suit her skills or outlook in any way, Sandra was struggling with self-esteem issues. By her own admission, her diet was poor, and she had stopped any form of physical training.

These problems were also compounded by Sandra's rheumatoid arthritis. This was causing her chronic pain and making what was already a difficult situation almost unbearable. Something needed to change.

Thankfully, Sandra found our program, and we were able to begin to address the underlying and fundamental causes of her difficulties. Central was inflammation. Sandra undoubtedly had a huge amount of internal inflammation that was seriously hampering her body. Getting on top of that was going to be critical to turning her health around.

One of the first things she did for her health was to cut out dairy completely. As we've been discussing in this chapter, that's massive for inflammation. Dairy consumption should be reduced as an absolute priority.

Sandra is now eating super clean. No fast food, no soft drinks, and carbs have been seriously cut. She also went completely organic. All the bad stuff has been eliminated and replaced with good, wholesome, nutritious food. The difference this has made in her life has been massive. Her whole mindset has improved, her self-esteem and self-confidence have soared, and she now has a job offer that she's very positive about.

Sandra found the workshops and community aspect of the program particularly valuable and has found that her motivation, sense of well-being, and overall health have all escalated rapidly. Sandra is definitely another success story from the six-week program, and one of which we're extremely proud.

Chapter Four

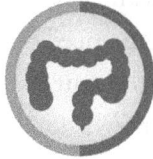

Gut Health
THE GOAL THIS WEEK (WEEK THREE):
To work toward healing the gut

- Improve the gut lining.

- Improve the health of your microbiome.

- Understand the damaging effects of antibiotics.

- Cleanse the gut of bad bacteria.

THE THIRD CRITICAL PILLAR OF YOUR OVERALL HEALTH PRO-GRAM SHOULD BE ENSURING THAT YOUR GUT IS IN GOOD SHAPE. This is a hidden part of overall body health, as the symptoms of an unhealthy gut often go undetected. Many of us don't even realize how common this condition can be.

I want to immediately reintroduce you to a concept that we touched upon earlier in the book: the leaky gut. In this chapter, we are going to fully address the leaky gut—what causes it, what can be done to avoid it, how to heal it, and a few actions that you can take immediately.

There is no doubt that the term *leaky gut* sounds slightly alarming! Well, it should, because it's something that you really want to avoid! Luckily, as always, our bodies are amazing machines, capable of rapidly healing themselves and overcoming any problems, so those of you suffering from leaky guts need not be overly concerned.

"All disease begins in the gut."—Hippocrates, the father of modern medicine, offered this wisdom over 2,000 years ago, and it has stood the test of time. If you follow this basic guidance, then you won't go wrong with your health.

Do something about your gut health. Trust me! Let's start with your steps to success.

YOUR STEPS TO SUCCESS

Step 1: Explore either making your own bone broth (see *Your Health Is Nonnegotiable Cookbook*) or purchase a healthy, organic, grass-finished, antibiotic-free bone broth in powdered form.

Step 2: Increase fermented foods and live cultures.

Step 3: Increase your intake of probiotics (high-fiber foods).

Tips:

- Stress can be a major cause of gut issues. Following a stress-management plan is imperative to both your health and the health of your microbiome. We dive deeper into this in the next chapter. Use the "Nonnegotiable Workbook" for the strategic tips we share with you in order to manage your stress daily.

- Managing emotions is imperative. Allowing negative, toxic, anger emotions to fester in your body can cause the deterioration of the gut and can have a tremendously negative impact on your organs as well. More on this to come when we discuss Chinese medicine.

- Remove products and stimulants that can aggravate your stomach lining and kill your healthy gut bacteria: alcohol, caffeine, unnecessary medications, smoking, dairy, gluten, sugars, vegetable oils, chemicals, toxins, pesticides, beauty products, skin creams, antibacterial soaps, and detergents and cleaning products (commercial soaps and other cleaning products often include toxic substances such as parabens, sulfates, triclosan, and unnatural fragrances; as we detox the body, these are definitely to be avoided).

- Make routine adjustments or potentially change your career. Workaholics and those who have stressful jobs, like police officers, stockbrokers, air-traffic controllers, night-shift workers, and flight attendants, can all suffer from a widespread list of gut problems because every day they are exposed to an influx of stress. This is due to the sympathetic nervous system, which produces a fight-or-flight response. When this occurs, a balanced lifestyle of the parasympathetic nervous system—rest and digest—is rarely achieved.

- Work hard to get antibiotics out of your life. Antibiotics kill your healthy gut bacteria as well as any harmful pathogens you were hoping to destroy. Doctors prescribe antibiotics far too quickly when natural healing processes can solve the root cause of the problem. Avoid dairy, as most all dairy that is not indicated otherwise is loaded with antibiotics. Be mindful of soaps that are antibacterial, as well as mouthwashes and toothpaste.

- Chew your food. Not only will it help your body better absorb the nutrients in the food, but it will also allow for easier break-down and digestion of the food so that it will pass smoother and quicker. The longer you chew your food, the more hydro-chloric acid is produced in the stomach to further digest and break down your food. In turn, this will aid in keeping your bowels clean. Food that sits in your bowels for an extended time is not healthy.

- Increase fermented vegetables and other probiotic foods. Probi-otics may help reverse leaky gut by enhancing the production of tight junction proteins that defend against intestinal permeabil-ity. Probiotics are microorganisms that possess health benefits. Indeed, probiotic comes from the Greek word *pro*, meaning "promoting," and *biotic*, meaning "life."

- Reduce the inflammation in your body by giving your gut a break. Fasting allows your gut to take a break from constantly working hard to break down and digest food. This is the best time to seal the gap junctions in your gut with bone broth. Bone broth has been known to help heal the lining of your gut. This can be equally true with the consumption of L-glutamine, which fuels your gut lining so it too can repair damaged cells and come back healthier.

- Dramatically reduce grains, legumes, rice, barley, rye, wheat, corn, soy, and the like to similarly reduce inflammation in the body caused by consuming these foods. These foods are loaded with antinutrients like lectins and phytates, which your diges-tive system simply can't handle, particularly when it is already in poor shape.

THE SCIENCE

Millions of people all over the world currently struggle with leaky guts, and the overwhelming majority of these have absolutely no idea of this whatsoever. It has been a principle of medicine for centuries that all disease begins in the gut, and a leaky gut can often be the root cause of numerous other health problems.

What is leaky gut?

A leaky gut occurs when holes appear in the tight junctions contained within the gut itself. This is often referred to by medical practitioners as intestinal permeability. This simply means that the intestine is open and porous, and things that are unwanted can thus pass or leak through, hence the term *leaky gut*.

Those people suffering from a leaky gut have usually developed a larger hole than is desirable in the intestinal walls. This means that things begin to leak from their guts into their bloodstreams, and this can result in highly intoxicating consequences. Naturally, the body does not react favorably to this occurrence and thus (as we learned in previous chapters) will recognize the foreign invaders and begin an immune or inflammatory reaction.

It is certainly common in modern medicine to address the organ where a particular problem emanates. Those with thyroid disease have their thyroid treated, those with a heart condition have those conditions addressed, and so on. However, this often fails to deal with the root cause of a particular issue or even numerous intertwined health problems.

Leaky gut really starts in the microbiome, so let's take a look at that as well.

What is my microbiome?

Microbiomes are not unique to human beings; indeed, they are found in all multicellular organisms. A microbiota is defined by Joshua Lederberg, professor-emeritus and Sackler Foundation Scholar at The Rockefeller University, as an "ecological community of commensal, symbiotic, and pathogenic microorganisms."

In the human body, this community of microorganisms is living within us at all times and plays a critical role in our health and well-being. Yet the microbiome has been relatively ignored until recently. Only now are we beginning to understand the importance of this critical system.

Microbes program the immune system, provide nutrients for cells, and prevent colonization by harmful bacteria and viruses. Thus, ensuring your microbiome is in good shape is absolutely central to your well-being, and poor gut health will inevitably result if it is not. We will be going into more detail on the microbiome in later chapters.

Why is the gut known as the second brain?

Increasingly, experts are referring to the gut as the "second brain." It generally comes as quite a surprise to learn that you have a brain in your stomach! But there is logic to this analogy. Although the "brain" in our gut doesn't possess the intellectual and computational ability of our more conventional brain, it does have a fundamental impact on our mood.

Of course, a poorly functioning gut will have a strong impact on the way you feel. That is quite obvious. But this goes much deeper than merely an upset stomach making you feel morose.

Our enteric nervous system is an incredibly complex lattice-like pattern of neurons which are scattered along the entire length of our digestive tracts. It causes numerous sensations within our bodies, such as butterflies caused by nervousness; thus, it plays a fundamental role in our psychological stress responses.

Around 90 percent of the cells involved in these responses carry information to the brain, as opposed to receiving it. This means that your gut can be as influential to your mood as your head, or arguably even more so.

Furthermore, as we're learning in this book and journey, bacteria play a major role in our digestive system, and the enteric nervous system mainly communicates with our internal bacteria. Estimates indicate that there are around 39 trillion bacterial cells in the human body,[1] and this staggering number alone indicates that this phenomenon will obviously have a massive influence on our overall health.

Our gut bacteria has developed with us since we were born, helping us to digest food and fight off foreign and dangerous entities such as viruses and molds. We need to ensure that our bacteria is kept both healthy and plentiful. When we fail to achieve this, the biomass of bacteria within us communicates with central neurotransmitters in our enteric nervous system. In short, it sends messages that negatively impact on our mood in order to make us address this bacterial deficit.[2]

Interestingly, studies have been published which indicate that those with healthy and diverse gut microbiomes are less likely to suffer from mental health conditions such as anxiety or depression.[3] Unfortunately, considering the unhealthy and unwise diets that many of us consume from a young age, we often do not have this healthy bacterial composition. When considering the rise in mental health difficulties and conditions, this aspect of human biology should definitely not be underestimated.

With this in mind, the term *probiotics* is becoming increasingly prominent. Probiotics nourish and promote your biome, being cultured with the strains of healthy bacteria. Yogurt is an excellent example of a cultured food as long as it's not the sugary, milk-ridden product that is now so common in supermarkets. Any yogurt that contains strains such as *Lactobacillus acidophilus* and *Bifidobacterium lactis* will greatly aid your bacterial makeup, along with your microbiome and ultimately your mood.

The relationship between gut-healthy food and our psychological condition is still being investigated, and there will no doubt be many breakthroughs in the years to come. As I mentioned previously, the science related to the microbiome is still in its infancy, as the microbiome was largely disregarded and discounted as a key aspect of human health until relatively recently.

Nonetheless, studies already suggest that a healthy gut can reduce inflammation and cortisol levels, lower your reaction to stress, improve memory, and even reduce neuroticism and social anxiety.[4] It seems inevitable that as more work is done on the microbiome, we will find it has even wider reaching consequences for human health than is already understood.

What causes leaky gut?

First, leaky gut can often be a genetic or inherited condition.[5] Most people in the Western world are probiotic deficient, meaning they don't have enough good bacteria in their guts. This is common in both North America and Europe; whereas people in other cultures and civilizations often having double the quantity of probiotics of Western dwellers.

A result of this is that people in the West are often missing micro-specific strains and types of probiotics that have a positive influence on our immune systems and natural digestive defenses. This means that children often do not inherit the ideal probiotic system from their parents, and this is then amplified by the way we treat disease in contemporary society.

Antibiotics Annihilation

How many people have heard of the term *antibiotics*? Hands up! Wow, everyone. Who would have thought it? Not that surprising, because we now use antibiotics relentlessly, in the Western world in particular. According to the Centers for Disease Control and Prevention (CDC):

- At least 30 percent of antibiotic courses prescribed in the outpatient setting are unnecessary, meaning that no antibiotic is needed at all. Total inappropriate antibiotic use (which includes unnecessary antibiotic use plus inappropriate antibiotic selection, dosing, and duration) may approach 50 percent of all outpatient antibiotic use.

- The number of antibiotic prescriptions written for children has decreased in recent years, but almost 30 percent of antibiotics prescribed to children are still unnecessary.

- Antibiotics cause one out of five emergency department visits for adverse drug events (ADEs). Antibiotics are the most frequent cause of ADEs leading to emergency department visits in children, and seven of the top ten drugs involved in ADEs leading to emergency room visits are antibiotics.

- We spent $10.7 billion on antibiotics in the United States in 2009, including $6.5 billion among patients who visit physician offices and $3.5 billion among hospitalized patients.[6]

In case you haven't guessed … we're taking too many antibiotics! Way too many! Antibiotics can have a disastrous and destructive impact on a person's gut. Meanwhile, the CDC also notes that "most of this unnecessary use is for acute respiratory conditions, such as colds, bronchitis, sore throats caused by viruses, and even some sinus and ear infections." These are exactly the sort of conditions that could be caused by leaky guts. So we're literally compounding the problem.

Then it's the usual thing that we've become increasingly familiar with by now: we get sick because of the drugs that we've been prescribed, so we go to the doctor to cure the problems created by the system, and then the system prescribes us with more drugs, medications such as nonsteroidal anti-inflammatory drugs, or sometimes even steroids. Those medications do not have a beneficial impact on the level of probiotics in the body. It just becomes a vicious circle.

Sweet Science

To compound things more, we lack probiotics in our diet. This isn't the case across the planet, but it is true in most of western Europe, and North America in particular. Eastern Europeans frequently eat yogurt and kefir; even Germans consume sauerkraut, although less than they did in the past. Africans eat amasai, and Indians regularly consume lassi. The Japanese have miso and natto. While yogurt certainly exists in the States and other Western locations, it is sadly not the yogurt that our parents consumed. So we're just missing out massively on probiotic food, while in many cases bombarding our systems with antibiotics.

Furthermore, we've discussed previously how unhealthy our diets tend to be in the contemporary climate and how we are consuming vast amounts of foods that cause inflammation. All of these things have a negative impact on the probiotic environment and contribute to an unhealthy gut and digestive system.

Eating excessive amounts of sugar can contribute to a leaky gut, as the sugar causes an imbalance of bacteria to the extent that it can cause yeast overgrowth.[7] Thus, yeast and candida begin to overtake and eject more important healthy microbes and probiotics that should be present within our systems. While some yeast is necessary and healthy, too much is detrimental, and the excess sugar that we are now consuming contributes to this.

Stevia can be used as a natural sweetener, while local, raw honey is also good. Aside from that, there's really no need for any added sweeteners to be utilized in your diet. Sugars or sweeteners should be derived from fruits and other natural products.

Oils and Dairy

Oils can also be a key contributor to a leaking gut, so you would be well advised to remove all hydrogenated oils from your diet. Remove soybean oil, canola oil, and any other of those bad fats completely out of your diet, as they will only cause inflammation throughout your entire body.

Dairy products don't help either, particularly the protein casein that is found in cow's milk. Unfortunately, this protein is also responsible for causing addiction to dairy products, especially cheese. Casein appears in a particularly rarefied form in cheese, and the substance releases casomorphins, an opiate, when digested. These casomorphins then cling to your brain, activating the opiate receptors, producing an effect not much different than heroin or morphine.[8] This is why you'll often find that people who go vegan find cheese the hardest food to give up.[9]

Grains and Gluten

Grains can also be a major driver of leaky gut, particularly gluten and phytic acid.[10] You have probably heard of the increasing number of people who are adopting gluten-free diets, with a notable example being the tennis player Novak Djokovic. Gluten is found primarily in wheat products, as well as other grain products such as barley and, in smaller amounts, rye. Wheat is also found in the majority of packaged foods sold in supermarkets.

Phytic acid is found in all grains, beans, and nuts and seeds. That doesn't mean you should view these foods as unhealthy, as in the appropriate quantity, phytic acid isn't unhealthy. The amount of the substance derived from grains can be reduced by preparing food properly.

Appropriately prepared grains, such as ancient sourdough bread or sprouted bread, can be considerably better than the sugar-laden bread that you will encounter in the supermarket. Quality bread is far less likely to bother people with gut issues, but even these are far from guaranteed to be problem-free.

Gluten is much harder to break down than other proteins[11] and can cause all sorts of unwanted health difficulties. When gluten leaks into the bloodstream, it causes endemic systemic inflammation,[12] even leading to autoimmune disease if it remains unchecked. So you should be particularly careful when consuming gluten. Grains and gluten are difficult to digest, so they should be consumed in moderation, at most.

Other Triggers

Another thing to avoid in order to reduce your chances of getting a leaky gut are GMO foods, but we've discussed this already! Try to eat local and organic; your stomach will thank you for it!

There are other possible triggers of a leaky gut as well. Emotional stress will often result in this condition, as will anger and other similar emotions. And those of us who had our gallbladders or thyroids removed,[13] or other major forms of surgery, are more susceptible to leaky gut. There isn't too much you can do about having had your thyroid removed, but you can be aware of your vulnerability. However, there is no doubt that addressing your diet is the best way to address a leaky gut and that this is the fastest route to a healthy digestive system.

So how do you know if you have a leaky gut? Well, thankfully there are several explicit symptoms that point to this condition.

What are the signs of a leaky gut?

It's possible to go into more detail on the physical processes associated with leaky gut, but here is a brief primer on what it represents and the seriousness of this condition.

The first major warning sign of leaky gut is any form of food sensitivity or allergy. You may have noticed that these are becoming increasingly prevalent, and the statistics on this matter are quite sobering. Researchers estimate that up to 15 million Americans have food allergies, including 5.9 million children under age 18. The CDC reports that the prevalence of food allergy in children increased by 50 percent between 1997 and 2011.[14] Guess why? Because more of us are developing leaky guts due to the toxic food environment.

Secondly, any form of basic gas or bloating can indicate a cramping of the stomach. Any digestive issues undoubtedly point to a leaky gut and suggest that reparative work is needed.

Strongly linked to the second indicator of leaky gut is the increasingly common inflammatory bowel disease, whether this takes the form of IBS, Crohn's disease, or ulcerative colitis. These all point to a particularly severe form of leaky gut and really should be addressed immediately. Chronic constipation and diarrhea would be other similar indicators, while loose stools are a telltale sign as well.

When considering leaky gut it is important to understand that it can lead directly to many other undesirable health conditions. Some of these are relatively minor, but can nonetheless be a warning that something major is developing. Food sensitivities, thyroid conditions, adrenal fatigue, joint pain, and headaches can all be signs that a leaky gut is developing.[15] Any sort of skin issue, like rosacea, psoriasis, even basic acne, can also be a sign of a leaky gut. Eventually, digestive problems, IBS, weight gain, syndrome X, even diabetes can be the ultimate outcome if leaky gut isn't addressed.

Some of the inflammatory reactions related to leaky gut can be quite severe, because we're referring to substances such as toxins, microbes, bad bacteria, and undigested food particles leaking into the bloodstream. Obviously, the body needs to protect itself against such substances, and thus some stronger immune responses can result. Many people are struggling with these immune responses right now, without even realizing it, and equally engaging in a reactive medicinal response that will never solve the problem.

Even some psychological conditions, such as anxiety, depression, and ADHD, have been linked with leaky gut, although these have not been entirely proven. While migraine headaches and muscle pain are also common for those suffering from the condition, leaky gut really is something to avoid.

Autoimmune Disease

A fourth symptom that can be attributed to leaky gut is an autoimmune disease. When the gut linings open up, unwanted proteins such as gluten and casein can leak into your bloodstream, causing the inflammation of your entire body. If this continues unaddressed for a long period, an autoimmune response will result, and this can lead to some disastrous consequences. Type 1 diabetes, rheumatoid arthritis, Graves' disease, lupus, fibromyalgia, and chronic fatigue are all potential long-term results of a problem that can ultimately be traced back to a leaky gut.

Thyroid Problems

Number five is thyroid and adrenal issues. Hypothyroidism, Hashimoto's disease, and adrenal fatigue are all massive warning signs that you are suffering from a leaky gut, as they are based on molecules that leak into your bloodstream, circulate, and once again cause that dreaded *i*-word: inflammation.

Joint pain and rheumatoid arthritis can also be strongly linked with a leaky gut, and these are also becoming more common in contemporary society. Rheumatoid arthritis is a chronic disease affecting over 1.3 million Americans and as much as 1 percent of the worldwide population.[16] Repairing your gut will enable you to heal your joint pain, and this must be one of the most convincing reasons to address a leaky gut.

Nutrient Malabsorption

The seventh symptom of leaky gut problems is any form of malabsorption issues. Any form of food deficiency, meaning that you are not extracting sufficient nutrients from the food you eat, can be evidence of a leaky gut. Most people in the Western world are deficient in vitamin B12, zinc, magnesium, and iron,[17] yet many of us do not even realize that this is the case. We have not been tested for them nor have they been taken into consideration in our daily diet. This problem is only amplified by failing to properly absorb vitamins and minerals.

Inflammatory Skin Conditions

Skin complaints can be another indicator of a leaky gut,[18] so any form of acne or rosacea should be seen as a warning sign. Dry flaking skin, eczema, and psoriasis are also common complaints associated with a damaged digestive system. The good news here is that healing your gut will result in your skin clearing up and your looking healthy and amazing rather rapidly.

Mental Health Issues

Finally, any mood issues or psychological problems can also be linked to a leaky gut. Obviously, this is the most contentious and complex area, as many factors can contribute to psychological difficulties. But issues such as anxiety, depression, bipolarity, ADHD, and even autism can be linked to an unsatisfactory digestive system caused by a leaky gut, and this makes perfect sense when you think about it. The link between mental health and physical health is well documented, and it is simply difficult to feel good if you are experiencing major physical discomfort and difficulties.

However, it needs to be said that the link between autism and a leaky gut certainly hasn't been scientifically proven. But worth mentioning is that there is no denial there is a psychological impact of having a poor digestive system. I am convinced that a leaky gut will have a much broader impact than we are aware of today.

Good Foods

So what should you be eating if you're suffering from a leaky gut? The first rule here is quite a simple one: stay away from packaged and processed foods. Don't even go down the supermarket aisles that contain such products. You should instead buy organically produced fruits, vegetables, sprouted nuts, seeds, meat, and fish, as well as fermented dairy products.

Even the healthier packaged foods are still somewhat processed, and not as easily recognizable by the body, which makes them more difficult to digest. You can bet your bottom dollar that anyone who consumes a great deal of processed food is suffering from a leaky gut.

The second aspect related to eating with the aim of eliminating a leaky gut really involves the fundamental principle of this entire book and health in general. Everyone's body is different. There are different triggers for different people with leaky gut, and some of them are going to be absolutely specific to you.

IGG Antibody Test

So one of the first things you can do ahead of addressing a leaky gut is to undergo an IGG antibody test. This will enable you to identify whether you have any form of food sensitivity, which is a great building block for eliminating your leaky gut in the longer term. There are absolutely no hard and fast rules here. You'll quite honestly find that different people have completely different food sensitivities. Lab testing is available, but you can also pick up home testing kits that will do the job.

So, for example, with regard to dairy products, many people respond considerably better to goat's milk than cow's milk. This is partly due to the lack of casein in goat's milk. But this by no means is universally true; some people experience absolutely no sensitivity to dairy whatsoever, while some may even experience a negative reaction to goat's milk. So don't take anything for granted.

In conclusion, there are, thankfully, four simple steps that you can take in order to reverse a leaky gut. Woohoo! Some good news, right?

First, remove any triggers that could cause a leaky gut, which, as mentioned previously, include substances such as gluten and sugar.

Second, replace these with foods with those that help to heal and repair the gut, such as bone broth and fermented foods.

Third, ensure that you include the appropriate supplements in your diet to assist the repairing of the gut—supplements which include digestive enzymes.

And fourth, it is essential to begin inoculating your gut and loading up with probiotics.

Supplements

Finally, I just want to mention some helpful supplements that will enable you to address a leaky gut. The first of these has already been discussed in this chapter, namely probiotics. But almost equally important is fiber, which enables probiotics to thrive in the body.[19] This means that a diet rich in high-fiber foods, such as chia seeds, sprouted flax seeds, and sprouted hemp seeds, can be considered particularly valuable.

Fiber can also be acquired via capsules of digestive enzyme supplements. These help your body to break down proteins, complex sugars, and starch, which are some of the most difficult substances to deal with.

The anti-inflammatory L-glutamine is a valuable anti-inflammatory and delivers some significant health benefits, including reparation of the gut and intestinal linings.[20] Two to five grams of L-glutamine powder can it be taken twice daily in order to derive this benefit.

Collagen powder, N-acetyl glucosamine, has also become particularly popular, even in mainstream medicine, as it plays a major role in protecting the lining of both the stomach and the intestines.[21] N-acetyl glucosamine also has a positive impact on osteoarthritis and inflammatory bowel disease,[22] making this a particularly valuable substance.

Quercetin is another substance that is not necessarily part of the North American lexicon; however, it also delivers massive health benefits. University of Maryland Medical Center researchers state that it is particularly effective at keeping inflammation under control. "Quercetin acts like an antihistamine and an anti-inflammatory and may help protect against heart disease and cancer. Quercetin can also help stabilize the cells that release histamine in the body and thereby have an anti-inflammatory [impact],"[23] a study from the university notes.

Quercetin hydrochloric acid is of critical importance in the digestive system, as it is the primary stomach acid responsible for the breakdown of protein in order for it to be predigested before entering the duodenum and intestines.[24] It is possible to consume this substance in capsule form, boosting your digestive and immune systems. However, guidance from medical professionals should be sought in this area, as tests are required in order to determine the amount of quercetin hydrochloric acid required. As always, this can differ from one person to another.

Massive Step

So . . . that was quite a lot to take in! Although I've tried to make the subjects as digestible as possible (we are talking about nutrition, after all!), it's also important to convey the science behind this topic. Sometimes this can get a little heavy, but I think it's critical to back up everything that is being said, particularly as these may be completely new concepts to many readers.

By the time you incorporate the guidelines outlined in these chapters so far into your lifestyle, you will have taken a massive step toward creating a new, healthier you. But don't rest on your laurels just yet! That's merely the first part of the process . . .

Challenger Story

Sabrina was a new member of the six-week challenge who had a clear goal from day one. She felt that she wanted to be a lot more active so that she could join her children during their physical activities.

Having had four children, life had just overtaken Sabrina's best intentions. She reached a point where she realized that she was missing out on so much. Sabrina was also struggling with a hip injury, which was hampering her efforts to improve her physical fitness and general health.

Sabrina explained to us when she joined the program or challenge that she had tried to work out in the past, but that it had always ended in her suffering from painful episodes. In particular, she had been through a hip operation, and this could be particularly troublesome. She also shared that she had tried several other programs, but none of them had produced the desired results.

That definitely changed as soon as Sabrina signed up for our unique six-week program. Her results have been quite spectacular: she lost 25 pounds over the 42 days and gained so many other physical benefits.

In particular, Sabrina noticed that her hair had more luster and that her nails were stronger than they had ever been before. Additionally, Sabrina had suffered from a raft of different skin complaints, but found that her healthy diet hugely improved the appearance of her skin.

Again, Sabrina cited the constant support and sense of community as being central to the reason that the six-week program worked for her. This is someone who tried numerous programs in the past, and none of them had produced the results that she desired. Yet Sabrina found that her transformation during our six-week program was beyond anything she'd hoped for and really represented a massive shift in her entire ethos and lifestyle.

Best of all, she commented that the changes she had to make haven't been hard. Changing her life completely hasn't been as challenging as she expected, yet her results have far exceeded her expectations. Sabrina is definitely one of our biggest success stories and an example of what can be achieved by making important lifestyle changes.

Chapter Five

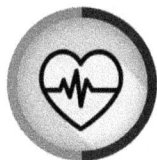

Stress

THE GOAL THIS WEEK (WEEK FOUR):

To Work Toward Cleansing And Detoxifying The Body

1. Learn the physiological response to stress in the body.

2. Understand the difference between healthy stress and deadly stress.

3. Help you build stress-management routines.

YOUR BODY IS THE BIGGEST ASSET THAT YOU WILL EVER BE GIVEN. It is the one thing in life that we can count on to always be there for us. Yet too often we completely fail to take adequate care of our bodies. Doesn't really make much sense, does it?

The hectic lifestyle that we tend to adopt in modern society inevitably leads us to place a great deal of stress on our bodies. I know this from personal experience, as when I began my journey as an entrepreneur, I put a huge amount of pressure on myself until

I suffered from burnout. I remember driving on a local bridge and reaching the point where I was experiencing panic attacks. Definitely not a nice feeling.

So before I go any further in this chapter on stress, I want to emphasize that I understand what it feels like. To be honest, I think most people do in this day and age. But we shouldn't surrender to this toxic environment and just accept that our bodies will be in a state of crisis. We should adopt a healthy lifestyle and mindset, and become all that we are capable of being.

YOUR STEPS TO SUCCESS

Step 1: You will need to spend a couple of days identifying your stressors. This will be explained further in the chapter.

Step 2: Start each morning with 15–30 minutes of practicing gratitude, listening to motivational material, and planning out your day.

Step 3: Transition from afternoon to evening (more on this coming up).

Step 4: Create your stress-remedy recipe (see essential oils, supplements, and routines) for the hacks.

At this point, I would just like to emphasize briefly that addressing this issue won't necessarily be easy. You will encounter challenges. You will encounter days when dealing with life will feel like a struggle. But nothing worth achieving is easy. If you want to improve your lifestyle, health, and general well-being, you have to accept that committing to this is a lifelong journey. It's about putting good things into your body and letting positive influences into your life, day after day, week after week, and ultimately year after year.

Sometimes your motivation will diminish, but the important thing is to accept this and push through it. Improving your body is a steady evolution, which requires you to make good choices, test your resolve, and evolve with the process as it unfolds. Only by committing yourself to this can you hope to achieve holistic health.

So we're all agreed that this is what we're going to do? Good!

Tips To Manage Stress

- **Identify Triggers:** Being able to identify the causes of stress in your life makes it easier to manage them. Once you know your stress triggers, you can identify which triggers can be removed or reduced. You can then focus more on coping mechanisms to manage the stressors you cannot change. Adopt healthy breathing strategies when you do notice stress building up; this can seriously reduce any problems.

- **Your Diet:** Your diet can make a massive difference to your mental health. A healthy, balanced diet rich in omega-3s, vegetables, and grass-fed, hormone free, antibiotic-free meats is essential for optimum health, both physical and mental.

- **Exercise Is A Must:** Exercise is great for both your physical and mental health. Exercise causes the brain to produce hormones called endorphins. These endorphins cause us to feel good and leave us feeling happy after exercise. In animal studies, physical activity caused the hippocampus to grow back to normal size after chronic stress caused it to shrivel.[1] Exercise has even been shown to be as effective as some medications at treating depression and anxiety.

- **Sleep Is A Must:** Sleep is vitally important for both physical and mental health. To have a better night's sleep, try to have a regular sleep routine—go to bed and wake up at roughly the same time each day. It's best to avoid screens like TVs, computers, and phones an hour or two before bed, and to use heavy curtains or a sleep mask to block out light when you're trying to get to sleep.

- **Do You Suffer From A Short Temper?:** Road rage is a classic example of the sort of temper loss that is ultimately driven by stress. Anger and irritability escalate rapidly if you allow yourself to be stressed, so if you feel this way a lot, then you should deem these to be telltale signs.

- **Identify Your Chemical Stressors:** Chemical stressors are any drugs that a person abuses, such as alcohol, nicotine, caffeine, or tranquilizers. It is critical to identify which, if any, of these substances you are overusing; this is the first step to rectifying the problem.

- **Benefits Of Having A Massage:** It's not surprising that we associate massage with the de-stressing process. Studies indicate that massage can lower your heart rate and blood pressure, relax your muscles, and increase the production of endorphins. Massage also results in serotonin and dopamine release, soothing you and making recovery from stress much easier.

- **Benefits Of Laughter:** Having a good old-fashioned belly laugh is another great way to counteract stress. Like massage, laughing triggers the release of "happy" chemicals, including NK cells, endorphins, serotonin, growth hormone, and interferon-gamma, along with a raft of other beneficial substances.

- **Benefits Of Sex:** Let's be honest, great sex is always beneficial! However, it can be an absolutely lethal stress killer, as well! Studies have shown that sex results in an elevated mood, while heart rate and cortisol levels can also benefit from intercourse. Sex can also be a good physical workout, and anything that gets the heart pumping and the endorphins flowing tends to be good for us and our mood.

- **Benefits Of Using Essential Oils:** There is a lot to learn about aromatherapy and essential oils. There are many essential oils available, and each one has different properties that can help relieve different issues you may be suffering from. Essential oils have calming, relaxing, and uplifting qualities that will get your state of mind back on the right track when you're stressed.

- **Benefits Of Music:** Music has been used for many centuries to elevate mood and restore harmony to the body, but scientific evidence has now also qualified and quantified this process. There is a huge amount of research available which demonstrates that music can play a major role in de-stressing our bodies.[2]

- **Benefits Of Nature Walks:** Getting into nature is just generally good for your soul. Connecting with the basic and natural elements of the planet has a massively positive benefit on your outlook. It's also good to get out of urban areas, away from the hustle and bustle, crowds, and pollution. Nature walks obviously keep your body active, which is always hugely positive. Nature walks are definitely among the top ways to handle stress.

Stress Management Techniques

So, along with having provided you with tips, here is a variety of stress-management techniques you can use in order to address the major problems in your life. Get into the routine of using these, and your mood will soon improve.

- Come home and go to your room.

- Your room should be your sanctuary.

- Use calming colors.

- Keep your environment clean and tidy.

- Ensure that your surroundings are decorated nicely.

- Ensure that your immediate environment smells nice.

- Open your windows for fresh air.

- Use a water fountain or negative ion generator.

- Lie on your bed.

- Close your eyes (use an eye mask).

- Use essential oils.

- Listen to your favorite calming music.

Experience a day-to-evening transition. Take out 10 minutes to do this. Transition between the hustle and bustle of daytime to nighttime.

Symptoms Of Stress

When you experience negative or unpleasant symptoms, this is your body's way of telling you that something is wrong. This absolutely applies to stress. If you're feeling stressed, then your body will respond accordingly, providing you with physical cues. So if you're feeling several of the following symptoms, then you could very well be suffering from stress.

- Difficulty sleeping

- Weight gain or weight loss

- Stomach pain

- Irritability

- Teeth grinding

- Panic attacks

- Headaches

- Difficulty concentrating

- Sweaty hands or feet

- Heartburn

- Excessive sleeping

- Social isolation

- Fatigue

- Nausea

- Feeling overwhelmed

- Obsessive or compulsive behaviors

BEST HERBS TO MANAGE STRESS

I'm a big believer in natural remedies, and there are some great herbal treatments that can help relieve stress in your body.

Benefits of Ginseng

Ginseng is a well-known herb, one that has a particularly strong anti-stress impact. Ginseng stimulates the central nervous system, lowering high blood pressure and increasing glucose levels. Studies in Asia on subjects with chronic fatigue found that the supplement improved energy and concentration while reducing anxiety.

Benefits of Ashwagandha

Ashwagandha is used in Ayurvedic herbalism due to its ability to regulate metabolic processes. Ayurvedic doctors consider this the single most important herb for men and women alike. Ashwagandha has been noted to reduce stress, with the substance also producing antioxidant activity in the brain. It is typically advisable to take 1 g of Ashwagandha on a daily basis.

Benefits of Schisandra

Schisandra is traditionally used in both Russian and Chinese medicine and has a particularly powerful ability to support adrenals, which lessens the negative effect of stress on the body. Interestingly, schisandra is also used to improve athletic performance.

Benefits of Holy Basil

Particularly common in British gardens, basil also plays a central role in the herbal medicine of the Asian subcontinent in particular. Holy basil can be taken in tea form and has a soothing effect on stressors impacting the body. It is an antioxidant that also results in reduced blood glucose levels when consumed.

Benefits of Rhodiola

Rhodiola is particularly used in eastern European countries such as Serbia and the Ukraine, which use an herbal tea brewed from the substance. Rhodiola root is renowned for helping people deal with physical stresses, and the substance also helps support the nervous system and overall immunity.

Standardized preparations are commonly used at doses of 100–300 mg, one to three times per day.

BEST ESSENTIAL OILS FOR STRESS

Essential oils are also great for relieving stress, so here is a rundown of some of the most beneficial substances in this area.

Lavender (*Lavandula angustifolia*)

Lavender is known for its adaptability and has performed particularly well in addressing both stress and anxiety. Research indicates that applying lavender topically may be the most effective way to experience its full benefits.

Rose (*Rosa damascena*)

Rose essential oil is rather powerful, and it requires only the smallest of dabs in order to deliver its full effects. Rose oil is known to evoke feelings of happiness, which helps reduce your overall stress level.

Vetiver (*Vetiveria zizanioides*)

Vetiver oil is notably interesting, as it is perfectly in balance with both the male and female anatomy. It raises testosterone levels in men, while producing a gentle estrogen-like effect in women. Known for balancing the female hormonal structure and reproductive system, this sedative is also excellent for calming your mood.

Ylang-ylang (*Cananga odorata*)

Ylang-ylang certainly has an especially unpronounceable name! But it is also notable for being particularly effective at dealing with anger-induced stress, bringing an immediate feeling of calmness and peace. Applying this substance topically typically derives the best results.

Bergamot (*Citrus bergamia*)

Bergamot has a refreshing lemon-like scent, but delivers practical benefits as well. The substance has been used during radiation treatments in order to reduce anxiety, and its stress-reducing properties are renowned. Several studies suggest that this is the best essential oil for dealing with highly stressful situations,[3] and the substance can be applied in a massage oil.

Chamomile (*Chamaemelum nobile*)

Most people are familiar with chamomile tea, and an explorative study conducted by the University of Pennsylvania School of Medicine found that the antidepressant activity in this substance is quite impressive. Researchers found that this essential oil "may provide a clinically meaningful antidepressant activity that occurs in addition to its previously observed anxiolytic activity."[4]

The National Center for Complementary and Integrative Health also found that chamomile can ease anxiety symptoms, and overall, the substance is enormously beneficial to those people suffering from high stress levels.

Frankincense (*Boswellia carteri* **or** *Boswellia sacra*)

This substance will always be associated with the birth of Jesus, but continues to have a positive impact in these modern times. Frankincense is rich in sesquiterpenes, molecular structures that can travel through the blood-brain barrier, and has a significant impact on both anxiety and depression.

BEST SUPPLEMENTS FOR STRESS

Supplements can also play a major role in the reduction of stress, and I particularly recommend the following:

Benefits of Phosphatidylserine

Phosphatidylserine is known to decrease cortisol, which can have a positive impact on the body's stress levels. A German study in 2012 demonstrated that, taken in supplemental form, phosphatidylserine "exerted stress-buffering effects."[5] Another study conducted by the University of Naples and focusing on exercise concluded that "phosphatidylserine may counteract stress-induced activation."[6]

Benefits of L-theanine

L-theanine is an amino acid that appears in high quantities in tea leaves. Evidence indicates that this substance is capable of stimulating alpha waves in your brain, which results in a relaxed state of mind, naturally reducing stress.

Benefits of Magnesium

Magnesium is another handy substance for addressing stress and actually tackles the debilitating condition in several ways. This shiny grey substance is able to stimulate GABA receptors in the brain. It also restricts the release of stress hormones, effectively acting as a filter to prevent them from entering the brain. Magnesium is so effective in achieving this that one study found that it is as successful as antidepressants in tackling depression.[7]

THE SCIENCE

I think that out of all the topics discussed in this book, stress is one that is most likely to affect us all. It is pretty much inevitable that you will end up in stressful situations sooner or later, and these will always have an impact on your anatomy. However, as I keep saying, everybody's body is different. You have to find an approach that works for you and accept that this may be different from what works for other people, both in terms of process and results.

Another concept that I'd like you to consider at this stage is that of having a foundation of beliefs. These can be the cornerstone of your approach to health, but should not be set in stone. Everything around us is constantly evolving, as is our understanding and level of knowledge. But if we eat something close to the way that we are designed to eat and move our bodies in the way that they are designed to move, we can make massive progress, even as scientific and human understanding is developing.

Dominating Our Diets

My guiding principle is that if something grows from the ground or has a mother, it is legitimate to eat it. Another way of putting this would be to have a motto of only eating food that's made out of food! You'd think that would be simple, wouldn't you?

Unfortunately, the majority of grocery store products are not edible! I know that's hard to believe, but it's true. Your body simply will not recognize these foods. Marketing has dominated our diets for over half a century, and the idea that we emotionally deserve treats is now ingrained in our culture. Hence the fact that snacking has become so prevalent, as we were discussing in a previous chapter.

Our unwise approach to diet has many side effects, one of them being aggravating our levels of stress. But there are many other issues also related to stress, and we will examine some of them in this chapter.

WHAT ARE THE DIFFERENT TYPES OF STRESS?

As I explained previously, although there is an anatomical justification for stress, too much is undoubtedly a bad thing. However, it is also important to understand that stress can occur and develop in different forms.

Type 1: Acute Stress

Acute stress is the most common type of stress among the general population, occurring over a short period. One of the aspects of acute stress that particularly characterizes it is that the source of this problem is always absolutely clear. Acute stress is triggered by obvious and immediate emotional and physical threats, essentially being placed in a distressing situation.

It is normal to experience acute stress, and sooner or later, absolutely every human being encounters it at some point in their lives. However, it can still become negative when acute stress is encountered with great regularity.

If acute stress occurs on a repetitive basis, then tension headaches, muscle problems, stomach irritation, rapid heart rate, and elevated blood pressure will be among the possible negative physical symptoms.

Relatively simple practices such as breathing exercises, meditation, and yoga can help ease the problems associated with acute stress, along with the other cures and medicinal substances already noted in this chapter.

Type 2: Episodic Stress

Episodic stress implies a longer and more enduring aspect to the stressful symptoms. Over a period of time, some people allow acute stress to become a regular part of their lives, and this is when episodic stress kicks in.

People experiencing episodic stress will have sensations of continually being on edge and will often be irritable and suffer from chronic fatigue. More serious health conditions such as migraines, chest pains, and prolonged depression can also result.

Episodic stress can be considered a significant psychological problem, and it should be addressed with a serious and sustained program of treatment. Unfortunately, many people suffering from episodic stress do not even realize that they have a problem, which is why, as I mentioned earlier, it is important to enhance your self-knowledge and be constantly aware of your mood and mindset.

Long-term episodic stress ultimately results in a higher risk of cardiovascular disease and mental illness and is definitely a condition to be avoided.

Type 3: Chronic Stress

Chronic stress results from enduring life circumstances which then perpetuate what is already a miserable situation. Long-term problems such as unhealthy relationships, poverty, and other debilitating life conditions eventually result in chronic stress. The condition will result when an individual can see no way out of a particularly stressful situation.

Chronic stress can lead to the most serious psychological conditions, including a higher risk of attempted suicide. The condition is also linked with:

- Lung disease

- Cardiovascular disease

- Hypertension

- Drug and alcohol dependence

- Some types of cancer

- Significant weight gain or weight loss

While much or all of the advice included in this chapter is extremely valuable to those suffering from chronic stress and can have a significant impact on their mood, it is also essential for people suffering from such conditions to seek therapy through a licensed counselor, psychologist, or psychiatrist.

STRESS IS CUMULATIVE

Long-term emotional stress builds up over time. For example, getting through a long, hard winter can result in this sort of stress. Any demanding situation in which emotional responses build steadily over a long time period results in this form of stress. Meanwhile, daily demands fluctuate depending on activity; in short, some days are more stressful than others. But obvious cues for this in the modern world would be experiences such as sitting in traffic jams, arguing with relatives, and work-related issues.

Of these three types of stress, long-term emotional stress is the worst kind, as it steadily eats away at you over time. Such major issues as divorce and bankruptcy contribute to this condition, and anyone who experiences this form of stress can become seriously fatigued over the months and even years that it lasts. This has a major impact on the body and basically results in the fact that you will never be in the physical, mental, emotional, and psychological state that you may wish to be.

STRESS AND YOUR IMMUNE SYSTEM

Almost everyone has encountered a person who is constantly struck down with irritating little illnesses like colds, coughs, and sore throats on a regular basis. Sometimes, sadly, that person is you! While there obviously can be a viral reason for such problems, levels of stress in the body can also be to blame.

Becoming ill after a stressful event is, in fact, to be expected. Your brain and immune system are in continual communication, meaning that psychological upset later manifests in physical symptoms. Chemical reactions triggered by stress result in the release of stress hormones, and these are rapidly pumped around the body. These then have the potential to interfere negatively with the immune system, resulting in inflammation, reduced white blood cells, and a higher susceptibility to infection and kidney damage.[8]

While this chemical reaction is part of our fight-or-flight response system, it can also have extremely negative reactions over a longer period. Prolonged stress can seriously damage the immune system, and this can have a massive impact on the well-being of an individual. Therefore, it is absolutely vital for your general state of mind and health that you address any symptoms of stress that you encounter.

STRESS AND YOUR ADRENAL GLANDS

Adrenaline occurs when we encounter an immediate threat. This shuts down our appetites, our sex drives, and ultimately our immune systems.[9] The physical process involved in this is the steroid hormone cortisol squeezing sugar out from our cells and into the bloodstream in order to provide energy so that you can run away from whatever is threatening you! Thankfully, we don't experience too many wild animals or dinosaurs in our contemporary society, but it's still important to understand this basic concept.

Adrenal Fatigue

Another condition that we should be aware of is adrenal fatigue. This is another stress-related condition that results in symptoms such as exhaustion, weakened immunity, sleep disturbances, and food cravings. It also makes your body a particularly strong candidate for inflammatory diseases,[10] and we know from our previous discussions how serious that can be.

In order to address adrenal fatigue, it is advisable to engage in various de-stressing activities. One of the best ways to kick-start this is to connect with nature, and this can even be achieved by simply doing a little gardening. Putting your hands in the earth, being surrounded by wildlife, and immersing yourself in the natural world in every respect is extremely therapeutic and can have a massively positive impact on your levels of stress.

STRESS AND YOUR SLEEP

We will cover the importance of sleep in the next chapter. But it may not come as a huge surprise to learn that stress can also prevent you from getting a good night's sleep. Indeed, the American Psychological Association found that 43 percent of adults in the United States indicate that stress causes them to lie awake at night. The same survey also found that 42 percent of adults reported a poor quality of sleep during stressful periods.[11] The risk of insomnia is also elevated by stressful episodes. The journal *Sleep* noted that the chances of experiencing insomnia increased by 19 percent for each additional stressor.[12]

When we sleep, our bodies switch from the active sympathetic nervous system to the calmer parasympathetic nervous system. However, stress interrupts this process, meaning that the sympathetic nervous system won't shut down effectively. This means that your brain stays in a hyperactive state, often leaving you wide awake well after bedtime. This is another critical reason to address the sources and symptoms of stress in your life.

STRESS AND YOUR SEX DRIVE

Stress also impacts another of the most enjoyable aspects of life, namely sex! Unfortunately, the hormonal impact of suffering from stressful episodes is quite negative for our libido. The cortisol produced by stress has the effect of suppressing our sex hormones, and a lower quantity of this substance results in a diminished libido.[13]

This is the most obvious impact of stress on our sex lives, but there can be more abstract influences as well. The emotional toll of stress can make us question both our relationships and partners, and this can actually have a knock-on impact on our sex lives, even if we are in a successful relationship.

STRESS AND YOUR WAISTLINE

Yes, stress can also make us fat! No sex, no sleep, overweight . . . are you beginning to see why you should avoid feelings of stress?

The avalanche of chemicals that are promulgated by a stressful episode has a big impact on our appetites. Adrenaline, CRH, and cortisol will flood through our bodies during times of stress, forcing our anatomies to respond to this threat by making us feel alert. This finally results in your body telling you that you need to replenish your food supply, as you have just caused the same chemical reactions inside yourself as would have occurred in ancient times when you scampered away from a wildebeest! Your body has been through a stressful episode and demands food for refueling.

Unfortunately, unlike those times from the dark depths of

history, we are often not running around all over the place, foraging for food—and ultimately survival—nowadays! We live in a much safer environment, but we create the same desire for food from sitting on the sofa and worrying about bills. So we don't burn anything up, while still creating the physical conditions in which our bodies demand a significant influx of calories, often in the form of fat and glucose. You don't need to be a nutritionist to guess that this tends to be bad for your weight!

Additionally, our bodies are supposed to store fat. Our ancestors' bodies were designed to hold on to these fat supplies for the long haul so that they could be used up in times of famine. Again, things have changed. We have an always-available food supply that is far greater—and more calorie, sugar, and fat packed—than at any other time in human history. This is the number-one reason why the level of obesity has gone through the roof in virtually every Western nation. The chemicals released in a stressful episode only compound this problem.

Thus, when we are stressed, we turn to unhealthy food. In the American Psychological Association's most recent "Stress in America" survey, nearly half of the respondents confessed to dealing with stress by scoffing indulgent food,[14] although it seems to me that the 40 percent figure procured by researchers is probably lower than the reality. I have seen so many people turn to comfort foods, such as ice cream, cookies, potato chips, burgers, fries, and pizza, as emotional support, and when you couple this with the overall obesity figures—40 percent of Americans are clinically obese,[15] while 61 percent of Canadians are overweight[16] (although larger percentages than this have also been recorded)—then I believe we can reasonably state that most people turn to food in times of stress.

There is also a precedent for this in the animal kingdom. A study conducted by the University of Pennsylvania showed that laboratory mice responded to stressful situations by eating more high-fat food pellets than normal feed.[17]

Stress is generally damaging to your body and state of being, but it can also incite you to eat in a way that is even worse for your health and waistline.

STRESS AND YOUR BLOOD PRESSURE

I would like to preface this particular section by pointing out that there is no hard scientific evidence which indicates that stress is a direct cause of long-term high blood pressure. But the two are strongly correlated. Possibly, stress contributes to other bad habits such as overeating, imbibing alcohol, and poor sleeping habits, and this then has a knock-on effect on blood pressure.

The risk of high blood pressure increases over time. But even short-term spikes in blood pressure can damage your blood vessels, heart, and kidneys. This is yet another reason to get a handle on your stress levels if they are veering into dangerous territory.

STRESS AND YOUR BRAIN

So how does stress impact our bodies? This can basically be broken down into four separate areas: cognitive, emotional, physical, and behavioral.

The cognitive impact of stress can vary in nature, but can include such sensations as loss of memory, concentration, and judgment.[18] Often we become too emotional when suffering from stress, and this can lead us to focus on the negative in every situation. Anxiety is also common, which can have a big impact on our potential. If we're always concerned about what could go wrong, which is an inevitable outcome of anxiety, we will never take the risks required to have a happy and successful existence.

Emotionally, stress probably most commonly results in a

short temper. A survey by the Mental Health Foundation in the UK found that 32 percent of people said they had a close friend or family member who had trouble controlling their anger,[19] most likely because we put ourselves under so much unnatural stress in contemporary society. Almost everyone has snapped at some point when they have felt particularly stressed. But feelings of being overwhelmed by life and an inability to relax, loneliness, trust issues, and a general state of moodiness are all common. Naturally, these are all aspects of our mindset that we should avoid.

STRESS AND YOUR MOOD

Modern scientific research demonstrates that stress is a contributing factor to a number of serious conditions. ADHD, anxiety, depression, and bipolar disorder can all be linked to high levels of stress.[20] Further research shows that stress can lead to cancer and heart disease,[21] underlining the importance of eliminating this debilitating condition from your existence.

Scientists now know that people with stressful jobs with few rewards have double the chance of suffering from depression.[22] This really isn't rocket science! If you hate your job, you in essence hate your life. So if you cannot change a job that you strongly dislike, it is imperative to identify a hobby or activity that you're passionate about in order to steer your cognitive processes in a better direction.

This is reflected in other parts of the world as well. Forty percent of European adults suffer from stress-related mental illnesses,[23] while in Canada it is estimated that depression will be the second biggest cause of disability by the end of the decade.[24]

Too many of us endure a rather joyless existence, and this far too often results in our attempting to anesthetize ourselves from the emotional pain involved. I know this, as I have done the same thing myself, too many times. This trend can be illustrated by the fact that

30 percent of US adults have had an alcohol problem,[25] while there are 22 million recreational drug users in the US as well.[26]

By allowing yourself to feel stressed, you are effectively missing out on life. Well, I'm giving you permission today to choose how you live your own life and what mindset you adopt. This is your choice, and it is important to understand that no one else cares! That might sound like a harsh statement, and I'm sure there are people in your life who do care about you, but they ultimately have to take responsibility for their own lives above anyone else's, and you should definitely resolve to do the same.

Only you live your own life, and you have to live with your body and emotions for every minute of every day. So isn't it about time you started prioritizing yourself over the needs of others?

Getting Hold of Your Emotions

There are many ways that you can mitigate the grip of stress, and thankfully, these are becoming increasingly well documented. Yoga and massage can have a major positive impact, while more Western people are engaging in the hugely beneficial practice of meditation. Listening to calming and relaxing music can also help relieve stress, and combining these approaches together can be really effective.

Additionally, as mentioned earlier, a wide variety of supplements are available that can help relieve stress. Combining the lifestyle elements with these herbal supplements can provide a powerful barrier to overcoming stress, no matter how demanding life may become.

STRESS AND BODY PAIN

Imagine yourself back in the world of cavemen and cavewomen. It is easy to say that life was very different back then, and the general environment contained considerably more immediate hazards than our society does today. When a bear is chasing after you, for example, your body is left with no time to digest food. This is quite obvious, and an equally obvious manifestation of stress. It is quite clear that having a bear pursue you will be stressful and that it will have physical consequences!

However, we often overlook less obvious manifestations of stress, yet exactly the same principles apply. Our digestive systems do not work anywhere near as well when they are being bombarded with stress and its by-products, and this has all sorts of negative consequences for our bodies.

Stress results in inflammation, irritable bowel syndrome, Crohn's disease, and many other undesirable problems.[27] This is due to a fight-or-flight response in our central nervous system, which effectively shuts down the usual pathways for digestion. The central nervous system also shuts down blood flow, which affects the contraction of abdominal muscles. Thus, stress prevents food from being digested effectively, which is obviously one of the most fundamental aspects of human well-being.

Stress also causes inflammation of the gastrointestinal system,[28] which absolutely makes you more susceptible to disease. Those of us suffering from poor digestion are far more likely to be constipated, while diarrhea is also rife among such individuals.

There are also some particularly alarming consequences of stress for your stomach. Stress leads to an increased risk of negative overgrowth of bacteria in your intestines.[29] This literally has the potential to eat away at your gut, and naturally enough, this isn't particularly good news for your digestion!

HIGH BLOOD SUGAR

Understanding the underlying processes involved in stress can be useful in seeing how it has a negative impact on our bodies. When we are stressed, the sugar in our cells is pumped into our bloodstream in order to provide energy to extricate ourselves from the situation.[30] But as we are increasingly sedentary in modern society, our bodies then have nowhere to go and nothing to do with this excess sugar production.

This inevitably leads to the excess sugar being stored as fat, which helps explain why it is more likely that you will be overweight when suffering from stress.[31] It's really important to remember that sucking sugar out from cells deprives the body of a key substance, and our anatomies still need sugar in order to make ATP from mitochondria.

ATP can be summed up as being the soldiers of power energy that are essential for any form of activity. If our cells don't have sufficient stores of glucose, then our bodies naturally crave sugar. Our anatomy is designed to continually crave sugar so that it arrives in our cells and can be converted into energy.

The Problem with Sugar

Unfortunately, there are two problems here. First, we increasingly seek sources of sugar that are considerably less natural and healthy than are ideal. Secondly, if we have excessive amounts of sugar floating around in our bloodstream, without being burned up, this will naturally turn into fat, and we will also be continually hungry, as our body will then crave yet more sugar.

This is a vicious cycle that will eventually result in our bodies becoming insulin resistant, so we will constantly have high blood sugar levels, as there is only so much that our pancreas can cope with. This horrible facet of modern behavior, a trap that too many of us fall into, eventually results in obesity and diabetes. So we shouldn't be at all surprised by the worldwide epidemic of these two major health issues.[32]

STRESS AND YOUR METABOLISM

While the two previous health conditions are both obviously important, the physical and behavioral impact of stress can be even more serious. The physical symptoms associated with excessive levels of stress are particularly debilitating, resulting in diarrhea, constipation, and nausea, all essentially emanating from stress in our bodies.[33] Stress also generally debilitates our immune systems, meaning that our bodies often don't even have the strength and ability to fight off common colds.[34]

Behavioral factors are also particularly significant, especially as many people will never associate them with stress in the first place. Sleep problems, isolation, agoraphobia, general procrastination, and the neglecting of responsibilities are all common for those suffering from excessive stress levels.[35] Sadly, we often make these worse by dabbling in alcohol, smoking, and recreational drugs, while SSRIs, antidepressants, and other forms of medication often exacerbate the situation as well.

I'm not here to tell you that you should never take any form of medication. That would be irresponsible. I accept that there are situations in which taking medication is necessary. However, I would also say that we are prescribed drugs far too readily and frequently. Before you pop any pills to deal with depression or other similar conditions, I would encourage you to try six months of proper nutrition and exercise, and see how you feel then.

We're going to go into this in the next chapter as well, but I'd like to briefly mention that sleep is the pinnacle of all issues. You need to sleep more than anything else in order to regenerate the cells in your body. Without sleep, you'll never fire on all cylinders, and you absolutely must respond to your body's natural demand for sleep. I will be discussing how to get better sleep, and its links with stress, in the next chapter, which is dedicated to sleep.

STRESS RELIEF

Another worthwhile activity that can really help address stress levels is scrapbooking. Looking back on happy memories can be very enjoyable and contribute to a positive mood, and the process can also be part of a creative and constructive project in your life.

Music also has a massive effect on mood, relieving stress rapidly. Playing soothing music can be particularly effective in diminishing the impact of stress, while even singing in the shower or while driving one's car can lead to a positive mood change. Experiencing stimulating music will release hormones that make you feel good, and doing this on a regular basis will have a surprisingly significant impact on your overall psychology.

FIGHTING BACK

Stress does far more than simply making us feel bad; it literally contributes to the destruction of our health and of our bodies. But we can fight back against this condition by adopting as many of the suggestions as possible contained in this chapter. There are also several foods that can help prevent blood sugar spikes.

Some foods that I would suggest in this area are as follows:

- Salmon

- Avocado

- Almonds, walnuts, and pistachios

- Dried beans

- Broccoli, cucumber, and carrots

- Cinnamon

- Apple cider vinegar

So take a deep breath and count to ten! We have to be aware of the dangers of excess stress, but there are strategies we can use in order to overcome the sometimes debilitating aspects of modern life. While our bodies are incredible machines, sometimes the culture and environment we live in today results in their natural mechanisms working against us. Unfortunately, this is the case with stress. But once we understand this, we can begin to take action, and a new and better version of ourselves will result.

We're definitely moving in the right direction now. You can give yourself a little pat on the back! In the next chapter, we will look at one of the most neglected aspects of modern life. So don't make that pat too big just yet . . .

Challenger Story

Kate Clare came to our six-week program after a particularly stressful episode in her life. As we have learned in this chapter, this can be one of the biggest barriers to achieving overall good health, and so Kate was certainly in need of a good spring cleaning!

Around three years ago, Kate's father passed away, a stressful enough episode in itself. But Kate was then also tasked with being the liquidator of the estate. Considerable family conflict ensued over this process.

The effects of this traumatic period took a while to sink in, as they often do, but Kate eventually found herself suffering quite severely from the symptoms of this stressful time in her life. Thankfully, Kate found our program through a neighbor and began to turn her health and life around.

By speaking to our stress mastermind, Kate began to understand the process that her body had been through. She also found that participating in a training program that didn't require her to travel to a gym on a daily basis was hugely beneficial.

Kate also made radical changes to her diet once she made a commitment to her health. She was able to cut out dairy and gluten completely and also eliminated all unhealthy sources of sugar. Her energy levels shot through the roof, and she began losing belly fat and massively reduced her bloating almost immediately.

It was important to Kate that she was able to significantly improve her health and diet, and be part of our community, which helped her enhance the well-being of her children. Kate placed particular emphasis on the community aspect, relishing the opportunity to connect with women who had been through similar things.

All the unhealthy food and habits were eliminated from Kate's life, and she looks forward to the future with an entirely new attitude, outlook, and joie de vivre.

Chapter Six

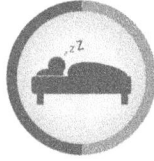

SLEEP

THE GOAL THIS WEEK (WEEK FIVE):

WE HAVE THREE PRIMARY GOALS IN

RELATION TO SLEEP:

1. To massively improve your sleep.

2. To create a powerful new sleeping ritual.

3. To educate you on the importance of sleep.

So we're going to begin this chapter by looking at your steps to sleeping success. Remember that you can personalize these steps by using your "Nonnegotiable Workbook."

Your Steps To Success

Step 1: Create a powerful sleeping ritual.

Step 2: Create a peaceful and calm sleeping environment.

Step 3: Use a sleeping mask and blackout curtains.

Step 4: Avoid technology three hours before sleeping.

Step 5: Avoid large meals three hours before sleep.

Step 6: Get plenty of sunlight during the day.

Step 7: Exercise.

Tips:
1. Make sleep a priority.

Sleep is absolutely fundamental to our well-being. This seems quite obvious, right? You don't exactly need to be Einstein in order to work that one out! Yet far too many of us neglect sleep. There just aren't enough hours in the day, so our busy lives take precedence instead. We think we can get by on a bare minimum amount of sleep, so it never becomes a priority in the way that it should.

Yet despite the fact that our bodies will inevitably encourage us to sleep if we fail to do so satisfactorily, many people do not realize just how important sleep is to their health. Studies have indicated that just one night of sleep deprivation can result in the body becoming as insulin resistant as someone suffering from type 2 diabetes. This translates directly to aging faster and storing more body fat than is ideal.

Far from being a trivial part of our overall health program, sleep should be considered the pinnacle of all issues. You need to sleep probably more than anything else, with the possible exception of taking in water. You must respond to your body's demand for sleep, at least if you hope to reach anything remotely close to your body's full potential. Don't neglect your sleeping time!

This should include ensuring that you get to bed at the right time in the first place. Simply sleeping at appropriate hours can make it easier to get to sleep and will also amplify the benefit of any sleep that you achieve. Scientific research indicates that human beings achieve the greatest amount of hormonal secretions and recovery by sleeping between the hours of 10 p.m. and 2 a.m. This will help rejuvenate your body and will definitely be positive for your general state of health.

2. Appreciate how valuable sleep is to your body, and honor your body by allowing it time to repair itself.

The amount of sleep required can vary from person to person due to genetics. Some people simply do not need as much rest as others. But seven to eight hours tends to be the norm. However, as always, it's important to listen to your body. You should feel energized, alert, and in good spirits most of the time if you are well rested and listening to your body's needs. If you don't feel this way, then you're not getting enough sleep, so act accordingly!

A simple way to address this is to alter your bedtime. Going to be bed earlier will help you to clock in those hours, as most of us fall into the routine of having a MUST wake-up time, but not a MUST bedtime.

3. Control your exposure to artificial light.

Exposure to artificial light at night, such as from laptops, TVs, phones, lamps—basically, anything that produces any form of light—is absolutely to be avoided. When preparing your bedroom for sleep, ask yourself a simple question: If you were to stand in a dark room without windows, what unnatural light would glow? Simply extinguish any such unnatural light.

Using red lightbulbs, candles, and shutting off technology within three hours of bedtime is the healthiest option. Some may not find this idea to be realistic, but you are in control of your priorities. You should also shut off any blue lights that may be present in your bedroom. Rest assured, you can dramatically improve your health by implementing a powerful sleep ritual.

In addition to shutting out light, you can also use blackout shades to make your room appear as dark as possible. Wearing an eye mask as you sleep can also help. I like to put two drops of essential oils on mine to really make the most of it.

You should also increase your exposure to natural light during the day. Not only will a nice brisk walk in the sunlight provide you with much-needed exercise, but 20 minutes of exposure to sunlight can increase your immune system and serotonin levels. Another idea is to buy a light machine that emits 10,000 lux of light and sit in front of it for 15 to 20 minutes on a daily basis. All of these practices can help balance your natural systems and make your body more inclined to go into sleep mode at the right time.

4. Move your body.

Exercise is key! Improved blood circulation, increased oxygen flow, and the endorphins that result from exercise can all make wonderful contributions to relieving stress and help you sleep better. Exercising at night is better than no exercise at all, but daytime exercise is recommended, particularly between 11 a.m. and 4 p.m.

In an ideal world, you don't want to spike cortisol too high in the morning or at night. If you are suffering from adrenal fatigue, exercising in the a.m. and p.m. hours is a no-no until you can heal yourself. But my first recommendation is to exercise whenever you can! Whether it's 6 a.m. or 8 p.m., move your body.

Sitting is the new smoking. Our bodies are not designed to sit at a desk all day, nor driving in a car or sitting on a couch. We were designed to be mobile and active throughout the day. Set an alarm to move your body at least once every hour. Every 20 minutes is ideal, but not always realistic.

Training and Sleep

Training can obviously have a massive impact on energy levels and can play a major role in achieving better quality and quantity of sleep. Equally, achieving optimum results in the gym is absolutely dependent on getting a decent sleep. So training really hard will help your sleep cycles, and sleeping really well will help your training performance.[1]

However, it is also important to train intelligently and appropriately. It is not enough to merely batter your body into submission in the gym; this has to be part of the overall natural cycle of your existence. Training should be done during the day and when your energy levels (if you're treating your body correctly) are at their highest. I recommend setting yourself a rule of never training after 5 p.m.

5. Optimize your sleep nutrition.

As you embark on this exciting new program, be open to experimenting. Try different approaches to eating before bed. Eat carbs before bed? Don't eat carbs before bed? I've read studies on both sides of that coin. You will have to listen to your own body on this one. Track your sleeping patterns with a smartwatch, see how fast and how deep you sleep. Do you feel antsy? Do you wake up in the night? Observe your own physical processes, and make adjustments accordingly.

It's also best to be neither overly full nor hungry when you go to bed. It can take a little bit of practice to get the balance right, but you will learn what works for your own body in time. Experimenting with macronutrient ratios is another worthwhile process that can help you get the sleep that your body needs.

Eating patterns

We have already reviewed intermittent fasting and the appropriate times to eat meals in previous chapters. But it should be emphasized at this point that eating food close to bedtime will naturally interrupt your ability to sleep.[2] The body automatically thinks that you are consuming food in order to turn this to energy and that this must be occurring so that you can undertake some physical activity. That would be a logical conclusion from your body, but we have now completely divorced eating from any such logical process!

So don't snack just before bedtime, and definitely keep the consumption of carbohydrates down to a bare minimum as you approach your sleeping time. Protein can be a good thing to eat before bed, as the amino acids in food containing high amounts of protein can actually be beneficial for sleep patterns.

6. Ditch the stimulants.

Although caffeine can have some health benefits, consuming caffeine after 3 p.m. can impact the quality of your sleep. The debate is strong on both sides of the coin as to whether you should consume caffeine at all.

However, when it comes to getting a proper night's sleep, you should know that caffeine excites the nervous system[3] and makes sleeping considerably more difficult. You definitely shouldn't consume any caffeine-related products in the evening. If your sleep doesn't improve while you're off caffeine, and it doesn't worsen when you start again, it's safe to assume that caffeine isn't an issue for you.

Alcohol Consumption

Before we get into this one, I'm not saying you can't drink alcohol ever again! I have no desire to become that unpopular! But do realize that alcohol can have a serious impact on your sleep patterns. Actually, the relationship between sleep and alcohol requires a little explanation.

Most people have heard of the concept of REM sleep by now, and it was further brought into public consciousness by the popular band of the same name. REM sleep, an acronym for rapid eye movement sleep, is a unique phase of sleep in mammals and birds, distinguishable by rapid movement of the eyes, accompanied by low muscle tone throughout the body and the propensity for the sleeper to dream vividly.

Memory processing is predominantly affected by different stages of REM sleep. And while studies indicate that alcohol enables us to fall asleep faster, REM sleep is significantly disturbed by alcohol in your system.[4] This means that you won't fall into the deeper levels of sleep and won't benefit from their restorative power. I will explain more about sleep cycles later in the chapter.

If you want to truly rejuvenate your body, then keep alcohol to a bare minimum, and pencil in an alcohol curfew alongside your caffeine curfew. I know . . . life is unfair, isn't it?

Sugar, medication, and smoking are other examples of stimulants that you should be looking to cut out during this program, and ideally in the much longer term as well. Of course, if you need to take medication, then you must do so, but what we're trying to do here is ensure that ailments which require medication go away for good.

7. Regulate your nervous system.

Managing your stress levels throughout the day can have a massively positive impact on your sleep patterns. Many of the tips in this book will actually help with this, as eating a healthy diet, getting plenty of exercise, and generally living a lifestyle intended to promote well-being will almost inevitably reduce stress levels. Practicing mindfulness is another highly regarded way to reduce stress.

Mindfulness can be described as the psychological approach of focusing on the present moment. This mindset can be developed through the practice of meditation and other training and is particularly associated with the Buddhist faith. However, it has become increasingly advocated as a mental health practice in the Western world in recent years and is definitely something that you should research and look into.

8. Learn how to meditate and control your heart rate.

The benefits of meditation cannot be underestimated, with the practice often being compared to a tonic that makes the body function at a higher level. It also has a profound impact on your overall state of mind. You should seriously contemplate including meditation in your daily schedule.

The effects of meditation are cumulative, meaning that they will increase over time. Several studies have indicated that meditation increases hormones and endorphins, and lowers stress hormones.[5] Meditation can even reduce the level of inflammation in our bodies, and as we know by now, inflammation is definitely something to be avoided.

Above all, the great thing about meditation is that it is completely free, yet it can kick-start our body and entire mindset in a way that few other practices and substances can hope to mimic.

9. Create an environment conducive to sleep.

In this technological age, there is a tendency to cram your bedroom full of stuff that detracts from the room's primary purpose. Only use your bedroom for two things: sleep and sex. That way you're making it a room with a positive intent.

This is the moment you've been waiting for . . . we're finally going to talk about sex! How can I put this subtly? Orgasm, orgasm, orgasm! Experiencing the state of orgasm acts as a genuine sedative for the majority of people, releasing hormones and endorphins that will result in an outstanding night's sleep.[6] Obviously, it is generally preferable to have another person involved in this process, but this won't have any impact on the positive sleep benefits.

You will find that orgasms are fairly enjoyable as well . . .

Make your bedroom a haven for sleep. You need to find a sweet spot that relaxes you, and this can include mood music, radio programs, and other relaxing material. It is important to emphasize that visual material on screen-based media should be avoided just before you go to sleep, and ideally after 7 p.m. each evening. This is difficult in a world in which we have become so screen addicted (don't get me started on this subject!), but it is certainly something you should aim for.

You should also remove all electronic devices from your bedroom. Yes, I know the temptation is always there to mount a television set on your wall so that you can watch TV 24/7. But televisions, laptops, cell phones—everything with a screen—is emitting radiation, which will disrupt your sleep. Reserve your entertainment for the entertainment area of your home, and keep the bedroom reserved for sleep.

Everything in your bedroom should be geared toward creating a relaxing environment that is ideal for sleeping. Even a compelling book can hook you and prevent you from sleeping as easily as would otherwise be the case. Make sure that your bed is as comfortable as possible, and if you're sensitive to noise, use earplugs to block out any external noises.

It is also important to regulate the temperature in your bedroom and keep it somewhat on the cool side. You may have noticed that you always feel warm in bed, even when it is cold outside of your covers. This is because your body's sleep cycles are subject to thermoregulation, which ensures that your body's core temperature is reduced in order to help you initiate sleep cycles.[7] The warmer the bedroom and environment are, the harder it will be for your body to achieve the ideal state for sleep.

10. Essential Oils and Supplements

There is a raft of essential oils and supplements that help support proper sleep, so I will go through a few of them here.

Valerian root helps increase the amount of the neurotransmitter GABA in the brain, which helps bring about relaxation and a general feeling of calmness. Drugs like Xanax and Valium increase GABA synthetically, but valerian is completely natural and safe. In one study, 44 percent reported perfect sleep and 89 percent reported improved sleep with valerian root.[8]

Passionflower is actually listed as a tranquilizing herb in Germany, and its calming, sleep-inducing effects have been known for a long time. It has a similar effect on anxiousness, so in combination with valerian root, it's a perfect way to slip into deep, restful sleep. Several studies show that it's an effective remedy for anxiety.

Lemon balm is particularly well studied. It encourages deeper and more restful sleep, as shown in a German sleep study. Additionally, it's an excellent antioxidant for the liver, a brain catalyst that helps improve memory, and a mood booster as well!

Hops is not just for beer. Studies show that those who drink non-alcoholic beer with hops actually experience improved sleep quality and reduced levels of anxiety. Hops has a lot in common with valerian root as far as their relaxing, calm-promoting effects are concerned, which makes the two a perfect combination.

Finally, chamomile is a sleep remedy as old as time. It's most commonly consumed in the form of tea, and its health benefits are incredible. It's an anti-inflammatory, helps with digestive issues, assists with skin irritation, is an excellent remedy for sore throats, and, of course, helps aid your sleep.[9]

Supplements that Support Proper Sleep

Magnesium is one of the most vital minerals when it comes to relaxation, sleep, and mental health. A magnesium deficiency can cause anxiety, sleep disorders, irritability, and abnormal heart rhythms.[10] The relaxing, sleep-boosting properties of magnesium are well known. One study shows that magnesium improves subjective measures of insomnia, sleep efficiency, sleep time, and sleep onset.

Furthermore, magnesium is a mineral that is important for relaxation. If calcium is the contraction mineral, then magnesium is the relaxation mineral. Magnesium is essential for countless activities in the body, such as energy metabolism, blood pressure regulation, blood sugar control, and regulating the central nervous system.[11] In one study, supplementing magnesium helped patients fall asleep faster and stay asleep longer. Foods rich in magnesium include seeds like pumpkin, sunflower and sesame seeds, leafy greens like spinach and Swiss chard, quinoa, black beans, and cashews.

Melatonin should also be a no-brainer for any sleep formula. Melatonin is the hormone made by your pineal gland that controls your sleep and wake cycles. Light affects melatonin production, and your body will naturally release more melatonin at night, which is why indoor lighting, TVs, and your cellphone's brightness can disrupt sleep. Melatonin causes drowsiness, lowers body temperature, and puts the body into sleep mode.

Made by the pineal gland in the brain, melatonin regulates sleep and wakefulness. The gut has been shown to contain 400 times more melatonin than the pineal gland, which emphasizes the importance of gut health for sleep regulation. When your body gets enough bright sunlight, this helps the body set its natural rhythm, referred to circadian rhythm. Melatonin's regular pattern increases at night because darkness stimulates melatonin.

There is something you can do to help regulate melatonin. Tryptophan is an amino acid, and melatonin is made from tryptophan in the body. So adding foods rich in tryptophan may help naturally raise melatonin. Tryptophan-rich foods include protein-rich foods like eggs, chicken, fish, tempeh, cheese, and oats.

The amino acid theanine also promotes a sense of calm and has many observable anti-anxiety properties.[12] Theanine is also able to deliver these rapidly, usually within 20 minutes. By reducing anxiety and stress, theanine helps quiet the mind before sleep.[13] Studies note that theanine improves overall sleep quality.

Kava kava, the national drink of the Asian nation of Fiji, delivers sedative properties and is commonly utilized to treat sleeplessness and fatigue, particularly in East Asia. However, you should also read up on the potentially negative side effects of this substance and make an informed decision about consuming it.[14]

Tools that Support a Proper Sleep Routine

Other tools that you might consider in order to support your sleep routine include:

Flux: this nifty program fixes your computer screen so that it adapts to the time of day and emits a level of light that is akin to the sun at that time. This prevents your body from thinking that it's 3 p.m. in the afternoon just before bed because you've been staring at a laptop screen.

Sleeping mask: studies have shown that wearing an eye mask reduces the time taken to fall asleep, increases sleep duration, and improves overall sleep quality.

Sun lamps: these positively impact your body's regulation of melatonin, helping you get to sleep and stay asleep.

Blackout curtains: these provide another simple but effective way of shutting out unwanted light.

The Science behind Sleep

So let's get into the science of sleeping. The last chapter dealt with stress and particularly the impact of cortisol, so this seems like a logical place to start.

Morning Malaise

One of the common experiences in our modern world that simply shouldn't be happening is the sensation of feeling very sluggish in the morning and then hyper later in the evening. I know that I don't always spring out of bed in the morning! We've all been there! However, although this may seem natural, it is a reversal of our natural polarity and indicates that our cortisol settings may have been reversed.

Cortisol is designed to provide a burst of energy in the morning;[15] it is effectively your "get up and go" mechanism. Unfortunately, for many of us, it seems that our get-up-and-go has got up and gone! When coupled with the fact that cortisol is also intended to help our bodies wind down in the evening, it is clear that the behavior, energy levels, and general sensations of many people are a mirror image of what they should be.

What Are Sleep Cycles?

You've probably heard someone refer to sleep cycles at some point during your life, but probably given the concept very little consideration. This scientific term refers to the way that human beings move through various states of sleep, with each sleep cycle lasting approximately 90 minutes. We actually experience five cycles during our night's sleep, with four of these involving non-rapid eye movement (NREM) sleep, and the fifth being when rapid eye movement (REM) sleep occurs.

During the NREM stages, we move from a very light sleep initially to a much deeper sleep by stage four. We have little muscle and eye activity during NREM sleep, but this changes during stage five. Once REM sleep kicks in, we experience short bursts of rapid eye movement. Dreaming also occurs during REM sleep, but our muscles are paralyzed during this intense bout of sleep.

So why are sleep cycles important? You may very well ask! As we begin to understand sleep more intimately, it becomes clear that not all sleep is equal and that waking during certain phases of our sleep cycles is recommended. Those who sleep well spend around 20 percent of the night in stage four, deep sleep, which has restorative properties for their bodies. If we don't get enough of this deep sleep, then we will feel drowsy during the day. A lack of deep sleep is also linked with serious illnesses such as diabetes, heart disease, cancer, and Alzheimer's.

If you wake up during the night, it's quite possible that you will spend an entire sleep cycle awake. This is due to your circadian clock, which we will come to in a second. So it is vital that you create the ideal conditions for sleep, get your melatonin to the right level, and get the rest that your body needs to function properly. Don't underestimate how important this is to your well-being.

How does the circadian rhythm affect my health?

Circadian Rhythms

You have probably heard of the expression *circadian rhythm* before. This is a natural biological process that provides an endogenous cycle over a 24-hour period, enabling the body to regulate behavior and make survival and elevated functioning more likely. Above all else, our circadian rhythms correlate with sunlight cycles, meaning that we should awake when the sun comes up and begin to get tired, and indeed sleep, when it disappears for the day.

When we fall asleep, our body switches from the active sympathetic nervous system to the parasympathetic nervous system. If this process is interrupted by stress, your parasympathetic nervous system will never shut down, and the brain will remain hyperactive. Lying awake at night will merely magnify problems and anxiety, so overall this is a counterproductive cycle to get into.

It is far too easy when suffering from insomnia to continually analyze your life at unsuitable hours of the day. It is very unusual to achieve anything particularly productive at 3 a.m., as we simply don't think clearly then. Luckily, there are things we can do in order to create an environment in our bedrooms that is conducive to successful sleep.

Early to Rise

This one goes hand in hand with the circadian rhythms that we mentioned earlier. It may seem counterintuitive, but one of the best things you can do in order to achieve premium sleep is to get up early. This links your endocrine system with the diurnal patterns of the earth.

You might find this tricky initially, but within a couple of weeks, or possibly even days for those with a particularly adaptive anatomy, your body will adapt to the new pattern of sleep, and you will begin feeling more refreshed and rested when you initially wake up. The sooner you get into this pattern, the sooner cortisol and melatonin will be released naturally and in appropriate quantities.

More to Learn

How is your body impacted if you don't sleep or if you have reduced sleeping hours? Well, maybe when you hear about the consequences of missing sleep, you will rethink your priorities.

The effects of sleep deprivation on the human body are far from trivial. It should be obvious that if we neglect to sleep, we will stumble through a great deal of our lives in something of a stupor. But so many of us pay no heed to this in our lives! It really doesn't make sense!

There are more serious impacts of a lack of sleep as well. Immune system failure, diabetes, cancer, obesity, depression, and memory loss can all result. Considering the extent to which we bombard our immune system in other ways, it is obvious that our health will suffer if we fail to sleep adequately.

As you can see, we already understand a huge amount about the impact of sleep, and lack of sleep, on the body. But there is a great deal more to understand about sleep. This is underlined by the fact that research into the precise functions of sleep is still ongoing. We do not yet know everything scientifically about sleep that it is possible to uncover, and no doubt there will be further health consequences of a lack of sleep that emerge as this research unfolds.

Nonetheless, we already do know a great deal about the positive benefits of sleeping satisfactorily. When we sleep, the majority of the body's systems are in an anabolic state, which has a restorative impact on the immune, skeletal, and muscular systems.[16] These are vital systems that help us maintain mood, memory, and cognitive function, and also play an overarching role in the function of the endocrine and immune systems. Overall, the mechanisms of satisfactory sleep are central to our well-being, and our bodies simply will not function well without it, or at least not optimally.

So it shouldn't be surprising that a study published in the *Canadian Medical Association Journal* indicated that sleep deprivation is directly related to an inability to lose weight.[17] Participants in an experiment conducted by academics were placed on an exercise and diet program, but those in the sleep deprivation group lost consistently less weight than the control group, which slept for eight hours.

Other studies point to sleep deprivation playing a major role in the development of cancer, Alzheimer's, and depression.[18] Sleep loss alters the normal functioning of attention and disrupts the ability to focus on environmental sensory input. Generally, being awake is catabolic (breaks you down) and sleep is anabolic (builds you up).[19]

Depriving Our Bodies

Lacking sleep essentially ensures that we are not firing on all cylinders. In short, it is definitely something to avoid, and going forward, I strongly believe that everyone reading this book should absolutely prioritize sleeping adequately.

However, if you're one of the unfortunate individuals who struggle with sleep, there are many things you can do to enhance the process. I want you to pay particular attention to these tips and tricks, as I know from personal experience that insomnia can be particularly troublesome and difficult to overcome. Meanwhile, many of us are simply neglecting sleep, which makes absolutely no sense whatsoever! Sorry, but it doesn't!

It comes down again to treating your body with respect and understanding that it is the most important asset in your life. I know I keep saying this, but hopefully, if I continue to repeat myself, the message will eventually sink in! The most fundamental principle is simply to truly understand, acknowledge, and accept the importance of sleep in your life and overall functioning as a human being.

Sleep-Stress Link

Another reason to prioritize sleep is that those of us who are unfortunate enough to suffer from insomnia are naturally more stressed than those of us who sleep adequately. Sleep is a break from stress, from all the worries and considerations in our existence, so it is essential to get a good night's sleep whenever possible.

When preparing your bedroom for sleep, another particularly worthwhile approach is to sprinkle lavender or other essential oils on your pillow. Let fresh air into your bedroom, and cultivate an environment that will be pleasant for sleeping. Melatonin is also an excellent supplement to use if you are experiencing sleeping problems,[20] although you must be careful not to use too much as this may have the reverse effect.

How Daylight Affects Sleep

When thinking about sleep, it is critical to get more sunlight during the day. As mentioned previously, melatonin is critical to your sleep cycle, being produced by the pineal gland in your brain and tasked with sending the signal to regulate the sleep cycle in your body. The production and secretion of melatonin are impacted by exposure to light, meaning that it is essential to expose yourself to sunlight on a regular basis. More light during the day and less light at night will add up to improved sleep.[21]

Get Grounded

Finally, this last piece of advice may seem a little out of left field, but it should actually be considered extremely valuable and constructive. As human beings, we are becoming increasingly disconnected from the earth and natural world. It is known scientifically that the earth itself is overflowing with free electrons of energy[22] and that these are transmitted to us when we come in contact with them. Several studies indicate that reductions in inflammation and pain can be achieved by getting in contact with the magnetic surface of the earth.

Additionally, it seems from both scientific research and anecdotal evidence that the earth's electromagnetic surface has the ability to sync with the internal clock of your body.[23] Your body is actually running on electromagnetic energy; heart monitors in hospitals are based on this electrical output.

So although this could seem farfetched to the uninitiated, getting your body in contact with the earth's electromagnetic field might be a game changer in improving your sleep. Try using earthing mats and sheets, which enable you to tap into the earth's energy within your own home. You might just find that it works wonders for your sleep.

Sleep Soundly

In conclusion, I hope this chapter has underlined why it is essential to sleep adequately and provided you with some food for thought on the subject. I also hope that the tips provided help you get to sleep if indeed this is problematic for you. Rest assured (no pun intended!), you cannot expect your body to function to its maximum potential if it is not rested and restored satisfactorily, and sleep is absolutely central to this process.

Okay, we're beginning to understand what is good for our bodies, so in the next chapter, we're going to look at what can be done in order to reverse the damage that our contemporary culture does to our anatomy and well-being. But before we move on to that, here is another inspiring Challenger Story from my six-week challenge program.

Challenger Story

Vanessa had definitely been through one of the most challenging life stories of everyone who signed up for the six-week program.

Her catalog of health difficulties began when she was pregnant with twins—challenging enough in itself! At eight weeks pregnant, it was discovered that Vanessa had a hematoma in her uterus. This solid swelling of clotted blood was obviously pretty serious, but things got worse from there.

Vanessa was hospitalized with hyperemesis and ended up on complete bed rest. She then went into labor at 20 weeks. This serious situation required a cerclage, a process that sews the cervix shut in order to keep the unborn babies inside the mother's body. Not a pleasant experience on either a physical or psychological level.

Because of this extraordinary situation, Vanessa was kept in bed for months. This had a very negative physical impact on her. She had neuropathy in her legs. She suffered from acid reflux. She even experienced shortness of breath while simply walking. In short, she wasn't in a good state.

Eventually, Vanessa connected with us via Facebook. This was undoubtedly an emotional time for her. She had been through an awful lot. It was essential for her to start with baby steps. While everyone's body is different, clearly her situation was particularly different.

But within just a few days, Vanessa was able to make massive changes. Her nutritional habits improved almost overnight. She mentioned that this wasn't even hard! Before, she would wolf down a whole tub of Häagen-Dazs in bed watching TV, but now she is eating clean and feeling so much better for it.

Vanessa has also managed to get into physical exercise, particularly enjoying the step classes that are part of the six-week program. She became a ball of energy in no time and has particularly benefited from the supportive community that helps keep her accountable.

In short, Vanessa has managed to turn her life around thanks to the help, support, education, information, lessons, and a healthy lifestyle that this unique program offers and represents.

Chapter Seven

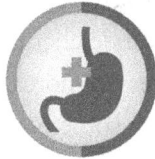

DETOX AND CLEANSE

THE GOAL THIS WEEK (WEEK SIX):

To Work Toward Cleansing And

Detoxifying The Body

1. Choose the cleansing or detox plan that will best suit you.

2. Educate you on cleansing and detox options, benefits, and precautions.

OKAY, SO WE'VE DISCUSSED SOME WAYS THAT YOU CAN CHANGE YOUR LIFESTYLE IN ORDER TO IMPROVE YOUR HEALTH AND START FEELING GOOD. That is all extremely valuable and worthwhile, but there is another elephant in the room that we need to address. Unfortunately, you've been filling your body with toxic material for several years, even decades. Don't feel too bad about it; virtually all of us do it. I've done it!

Luckily, it is possible to undo a lot of the damage by engaging in a detox and cleansing process. A seven-day juice cleanse is a wonderful way to aid your health transformation and will make it easier to keep your body on track in the future. When you feed your body nothing but wholesome, raw food for an entire week, you effectively flush out your entire system. You're really giving yourself an excellent foundation to make all the health and lifestyle changes your body needs.

We will go into this process in more depth in the next chapter, but first I'd like to discuss with you some benefits of detoxing completely. I'm sure some of you will feel somewhat dubious about eating no solid foods for an entire week. That is an entirely natural reaction. But you don't actually need solid foods in order to survive, and indeed prosper. This is a psychological trick that is played on us by our bodies. Our bodies are super smart, and the bacteria and microbes living within them know exactly how to get what they want!

There are some practical aspects of the process that you need to understand if you are to get the most out of it. I definitely want everyone who reads this book to participate in this juicing program, as I know it will make you all feel absolutely fantastic! You can't afford to not try it, particularly if you've been experiencing health issues.

But we'll go into that in more depth later on. We're going to start by outlining your steps to success in this detox process.

YOUR STEPS TO SUCCESS

Step 1: Prepare for your cleanse or detox the week before by increasing fasting windows, reducing carbs, and sticking to fruits, vegetables, nuts, and seeds. Cut out dairy, gluten, and processed foods, while limiting proteins and any stimulants such as alcohol, caffeine, sugar, and smoking.

Step 2: Plan your recipes well in advance. But . . . you cannot prep your foods. Juices should be consumed at the time that you squeeze them. Have all of your stock ready and organized so that you know exactly what you are doing. Don't wing it! Consult our *Your Health Is Nonnegotiable Cookbook* and workbook for additional planning tools and recipes.

Step 3: Choose a week that is not overly stressful and a time in your life when you are not in a state of hardship. The body needs its time to heal and repair in a somewhat mindful state.

Step 4: Plan your workouts in advance and listen to your body. You can plan to go lighter on the load this week. Include yoga and meditation with mild weight training, alongside endurance training. I would not engage in any HIIT training during this week.

Tips:
Is Your Body Toxic? Do You Need A Detox?

If you're suffering from any of the following symptoms, then you would probably benefit from a detox:

- Constipation

- Gas and bloating

- Headaches

- White tongue or bad breath (Candida)

- Fatigue

- Aches and pains

- Belly fat

- Skin problems

- Food craving

- Mood swings

- Weight loss resistance

- Acne

- Body odor

- Dark circles under the eyes

BENEFITS OF DOING A DETOX

Cleanses the Liver

Detox and cleansing will also improve the way your liver functions,[1] which will be particularly beneficial considering the amount of stress many of us place on this vital organ. Hopefully, you don't drink excessively, but many people's alcohol consumption makes the liver work even harder. This is extremely bad for our bodies, as the liver is our main detoxification organ and plays an absolutely central role in the proper functioning of the body. Every single molecule of nutrition absorbed through the intestinal wall is eventually detoxified in this key organ.

Unfortunately, in our crazy modern world, we fill our bodies with so many toxins that our livers struggle to cope. Again, the miracle of the human body is that it is incredibly self-sustaining, and the liver is able to regenerate itself even when it has been badly damaged.[2] Detoxing and cleansing will reduce the load imposed on your liver, improving its functioning in the future. I cannot overstate how important this is for your health and well-being.

Balances Hormones

Many people, women, in particular, experience hormonal problems in life. This is far from helped by the unhealthy eating habits that many of us have developed. Detoxing effectively enables us to push the reset button on our body and rebalance our hormonal structure.

If you're struggling with a hormonal imbalance, you may encounter some of the following symptoms:

- Low energy, dragging yourself in the afternoon, feeling sluggish

- Mood swings, depression, anxiety, irritability, weepiness

- Painful, heavy, or irregular periods

- Breast tenderness

- Bloating

- Acne, rashes, dry skin

- Weight gain

- Low libido

- Vaginal dryness

- Hot flashes and night sweats

- Infertility or miscarriage

- Ovarian cysts or uterine fibroids

- Endometriosis

- Hair loss or excess body hair

- Muscle aches, joint pain

- Estrogen dominance

If any of these apply to you, detoxing can help you rectify the situation.

Clears Inflammation in the Body

Yes, it's that *i*-word again! Inflammation, inflammation, inflammation! Everywhere you look in the human body, you will find inflammation. That is just a by-product of our contemporary culture. The situation is only going to improve when our diets and lifestyles improve. We have already gone over all of the worrying conditions that are associated with inflammation in the body, so anything that aids with reducing this process must be considered positive.

A cleanse and detox program with juices and smoothies will indeed help the body fight inflammation and vastly improve your overall anatomical health.[3] Meanwhile, issues such as headaches, skin rashes, general aches and pains, bloating, and trapped gas will all markedly improve as a direct result of this nutritional approach.[4]

Helps People Who Are Dealing with an "-itis"

Many "-itis" conditions—allergies, maladies, and general dysfunction in the body—often result in medics treating the symptoms rather than the cause. In many cases, the cause is the toxic crap that we put into our bodies. By detoxing and cleansing our bodies, many people who previously experienced often debilitating medical conditions find that they rapidly dissipate as a direct consequence.

Creating New Cartilage Helps the Body Heal and Repair Faster

Some positive impacts of detox and cleansing would be extremely difficult for the uninitiated to predict. One such impact is the ability of detox to help the body create new cartilage, with the knock-on effect of healing and repairing your anatomy more quickly. Cartilage is a particularly important part of the body, as it works like a cushion, protecting bones and joints during movement. This is obviously important for anyone intending to lead an active lifestyle, as we all should.

As we get older, it is important to look after our cartilage because it begins to break down and become less spongy over time. This can lead to friction and pain in our joints, a condition referred to as osteoarthritis. While doctors will recommend painkillers and supplements for such problems, a detox diet can also set you on the right road to managing your condition and even building new cartilage.

The University of Maryland Medical Center recommends an anti-inflammatory diet to help prevent and manage osteoarthritis.[5] Step one in this process is to detox the body in order to repair the damage that has been done previously and press the reset button. The inflammation chapter provides further information on foods that you may wish to eat as well as those to avoid in order to help with this issue.

Weight Loss

Those individuals carrying excess weight can certainly expect to lose at least some of it on a juicing program. Some of this will be water weight, but fat will also dissipate as well. Another benefit of detoxing and cleansing is that some undesirable physical symptoms that you have experienced previously will diminish, or possibly disappear. Detoxing will enable you to reduce your stored belly fat, making you both look and feel better.

Healthier Skin

Oxygen is also required in order to activate the skin, providing a second elimination channel for any unwanted and unrequired substances. So it is important to get outside three to four times per day and get some sun, as this will really get your whole system moving and also contribute positively to your physical appearance.

Reduce Aging

Detox and cleansing can also play a part in reducing the aging process, leaving you looking and feeling younger and more vibrant. The busy lives that we lead today almost inevitably create stress, which can result in our bodies aging more rapidly than they should. Additionally, the overindulgence and generally poor dietary practices many people engage in put unnecessary strain on our anatomies. One thing affected by this is the tone and elasticity of the skin. This naturally results in premature aging and wrinkles.

Many people also discount the fact that the skin plays a critical role in detoxification; in fact, it is the second most important organ after the liver in this regard.[6] Anything that your liver is unable to handle is effectively transported to the skin, resulting in spots, dull skin, wrinkles, and eye bags. But by engaging in a detox and cleansing plan, you begin to rejuvenate your skin and reverse this process.

Detoxification will help your body remove toxins while absorbing the antioxidants found in the healthy foods you will be eating during this period, which will be hugely beneficial. These protect your skin against such aging components as UV light, pollution, sugar, smoking, and fried and processed foods.[7]

Rashes

Although detoxing is excellent news for the skin, it is worth mentioning that in the longer term, your body rids itself of the unwanted substances that it has been toiling against for quite some time. This is no cause for alarm and will pass in due course.

However, it is also advisable to avoid chemicals contained in certain cosmetic products during the process (and, ideally, on a permanent basis). These include sodium lauryl sulfate, which is found in most soaps; propylene glycol, which is commonly found in cosmetics; and synthetic fragrances.

Removes Metals

Many chronic problems in the body actually emanate from metallic elements. Such symptoms as fatigue, migraine headaches, joint pain, brain fog, general sluggishness, and many others are ultimately caused by metal within the body. These symptoms can persist for many years, or even decades, despite the intervention of healthcare professionals, as every issue other than the metallic elements within your anatomy are addressed unsuccessfully.

The modern world bombards us with toxins of every conceivable nature. We are subjected to a daily onslaught of unsuitable chemicals from such sources as a pollution, plastics, industrial cleaning agents, and chemicalized food. That is to say nothing of the thousands of chemicals that are introduced into the environment on a daily basis. If you are experiencing problems with your body, toxic heavy metals could well be to blame.

Heavy-metal toxicity is derived from such substances as mercury, aluminum, copper, cadmium, nickel, and lead. This undoubtedly represents one of the greatest threats to our overall health and well-being. Heavy-metal toxicity is incredibly common, yet it is rarely diagnosed by the medical establishment. It hides inside our bodies, never being discovered unless it is actively sought.

Consequently, many of us are carrying around metal inside of us, which is doing our bodies absolutely no good whatsoever. Such substances can promote inflammation in the digestive tract and release poisons into our system. Heavy metals can also be a source of food for viruses, bacteria, parasites, and other pathogens. This can obviously lead to a raft of symptoms so numerous that it is literally impossible to list them all. But above all else, our bodies can become overrun with bacteria, which is extremely bad news for their general functioning.

Juice detoxing is an effective way of beginning to flush out these unwanted heavy-metal invaders and taking control of your internal systems once more.[8] This is highly recommended, since in our contemporary chemically infused climate, many of us are living with a metallic interior without ever knowing it.

Mental Clarity

Many people nowadays find themselves increasingly fatigued, distracted, and moody. This set of symptoms is often described as brain fog, a catchall term for our mental faculties working at less than their premium level. Brain fog is now a common symptom of the advanced industrialized society that we live in, which has produced many poisonous products and by-products, not least the processed, chemicalized, often factory-produced foods that we eat today.

This means that many of us suffer from nutrient deficiencies, excessive sugar consumption, sleep deficit, poor energy levels, and many other things that we are addressing in this book. This can lead to the aforementioned brain fog. Our brains rely on a continual stream of vitamins and minerals, amino acids, essential fatty acids, and glucose, along with sufficient rest, and when this balance is off-kilter, it responds unfavorably!

Researchers from the departments of physiology and medicine at New York Medical College in Valhalla define brain fog as "an interaction of physiological, cognitive, and perceptual factors."[9] It can include low energy or fatigue, irritability, trouble concentrating, headaches, forgetfulness, and trouble remembering information, low motivation, feeling hopeless or mildly depressed, anxiety, confusion, trouble sleeping through the night or insomnia, and difficulty exercising.

Detoxing helps us break down brain fog by ridding our internal systems of the toxic substances that have been ailing them and giving them what they do need instead. Over a period of time, this will help to ease and then eradicate brain fog, enabling you to think more clearly and operate more effectively.

Depression, anxiety, and panic attacks are some other symptoms that can be addressed by detoxing.[10] Overall, the detox and cleanse process will clear your thought processes and get you firing on all cylinders again.

Addiction Habits

Detox and cleanse can also help you quit several painful addiction habits that can hinder you in life. It has actually been known for people to quit dangerous alcohol habits after a program of fasting and juicing. The detox program will also help you with a wide variety of food addictions. By denying your body the harmful things that you've become dependent on, you can help snap those addictions and build a brand-new you.

Another benefit of the juicing program outlined in this book is that it can play a role in reducing your susceptibility toward some extremely serious mental conditions. Many people's diets are hindering their immune systems, with the liver particularly being hampered. When the liver is poisoned, the lactate from cancer cells can backwash into the lymph and blood systems, and this is a serious cancer risk.[11] Detoxing helps turn the tide on this issue, potentially adding years to your life and preventing a lot of unnecessary suffering.

Tumor Reduction

Detoxing can also play a role in reducing tumors in the body. When you eat, the level of white blood cells in your body increases. This can potentially increase the size of tumors contained within your anatomy. However, when your immune system is overburdened with poisonous toxins to break down, it is not able to destroy these tumors.[12] This means that fasting and detox can really help reduce your chances of developing a nasty tumor.

Before we get into the science of detox, I just want to go over a few more aspects of detoxing and cleansing in list form so that you have some key information on hand at all times.

The Most Toxic Foods

Dairy

Corn

Soy

Shellfish

Gluten

Alcohol

Processed foods

Sugar

Best Herbs To Detox

Mint

Ginger = Detoxes the gut

Rosemary = Detoxes the adrenals and kidneys

Dandelion = Detoxes the liver

Cinnamon = #1 antioxidant; fat soluble; #1 for diabetes; balances blood sugar levels

Cayenne pepper = Detoxes the blood

Best Foods To Detox

Watermelon = Helps with fluid exchange; cleans out the cells

Cucumber = Helps with fluid exchange; cleans out the cells

Lemon = Detoxes the liver

Lime = Detoxes the liver

Grapefruit = Detoxes the liver

Berries = Benefit the kidneys and adrenals

Best Essential Oils To Detox

Orange oil = Detoxes the liver and your entire lymphatic system

Rosemary oil = Detoxes adrenals and kidneys

Turmeric oil = Detoxes the liver and kidneys

Vetiver = Improves brain functioning

Black pepper oil = Detoxes your cardiovascular system

Additional Practices

Intermittent fasting (water fast)

Shinrin-yoko

Meditation and yoga

Eliminate meats and dairy

Benefits Of Detox And Cleanses

Heavy on veggies/Light on fruit

Detoxification

Mental clarity

Reduces inflammation

Reduction in craving

Weight loss

Types Of Detox And Cleanses

Water fast

Juice cleanse

Bone broth cleanse

Daniel diet (raw food, fruit, nuts, seeds only)

Mono diet (eat only one thing)

Intermittent fasting

Pros Of Juicing

Easily digestible

Easy to consume

Easy to absorb nutrients

Aids in cellular regeneration

Can be high in sugars with fruits, so stick to vegetables

Cons Of Juicing

Doesn't achieve weight loss

Too much sugar

Missing out on fiber with too much sugar

Ease into juicing; reduce sugar, carbs, processed foods, and addictive stimulants at least a week in advance

Great Detox Drink

Apple cider vinegar = Full of enzymes, good bacteria; burns fat; drops blood sugar levels

Lemon juice and cinnamon = #1 antioxidant; fat soluble; #1 for diabetes; balances blood sugar levels

Cayenne pepper = Drops blood pressure

A few drops of honey

THE SCIENCE

So let's get into the science of detox. While we've already gone over quite a few reasons why you should consider detoxing, I'd like to begin this section be reiterating the benefits of cleansing.

Why Do a Cleanse?

First, by detoxing and cleansing you are giving your stomach a break, for which it will be eternally grateful! It has more than likely been bombarded with crap for many years, and both your gut and digestive systems have received something of an onslaught. It is the miracle of the human anatomy that the systems and organs inside us will keep us going even while we're doing this. But can they maintain optimum health when being fed so inappropriately? You can bet your bottom dollar that they cannot!

Statistics indicate that approximately one-third of all Americans suffer from stomach problems such as acid reflux. Sixty million Americans alone report getting heartburn.[13] Consequently, millions of people all across North America, and for that matter, the Western world as a whole, are taking acid-suppressing drugs in an attempt to alleviate symptoms. Of course, as we've discussed previously, the medics who prescribe these drugs have never been trained in nutrition and are also trained to push drugs on people. There are lots of good people who are doctors, but that's just the truth.

Stomach acids are actually required by the body,[14] so suppressing them is not necessarily a good thing, let alone doing so with medication. By engaging in a seven-day juice cleanse, your stomach is required to continually extract nutrients, and due to the digestion and processing necessitated by such processes as churning, acid and digestive enzyme production is reduced. Effectively, you are giving your stomach a little vacation! It probably deserves one after all these years of toxic eating!

Repairing the Gut

The overwhelming majority of people have gut difficulty, regardless of whether they realize this or not. This is almost inevitable considering the foods that we put into our bodies on a daily basis, along with the accompaniment of chemicalized ingredients, herbicides, pesticides, etc. Other food groups such as saturated fats, refined processed carbs, foods with additives, allergenic foods, and components of food such as bad bacteria, yeast, fungi, and parasites can also put a strain on the stomach.

All of this leads to an imbalance in the gut microbiome, and any form of imbalance in the body is not a good thing! Recently, the neuroscientist John Cryan, a professor at University College Cork in Ireland, has engaged in groundbreaking research,[15] which he suggests points to the microbiome being far more significant than was previously understood or supposed.

Cryan and his team performed experiments with mice and found that brain development and behavior could be directly impacted by their microbiome being inadequately aligned. "In these mice, the brains don't develop properly," Cyan explained. "Their nerve cells don't talk to each other appropriately, thus implicating the microbiome in a variety of disorders. . . . We've also shown changes in anxiety behavior, fear behavior, learning, stress response, the blood-brain barrier. We found a deficit in social behavior, so for social interactions, we have an appropriate repertoire of bacteria in the gut as well."[16]

Naturally, this could also have a major impact on humans, and Cryan believes that reforming the microbiome is the absolute key to human health in a wide variety of areas. So flushing the gut out with a seven-day juice cleanse is hugely beneficial. It can also help mend the intestinal wall barrier and help prevent leaky gut syndrome,[17] which you may remember from previous chapters. Consuming a micro- and phytonutrient-dense raw juice diet will enable your intestinal tract to more readily absorb nutrients, kick-starting your entire digestive system and getting your gut back on track.[18]

Appetite Reduction

Other systems and organs within your body will also benefit from detoxing and cleansing. Juicing doesn't reduce the size of your stomach, but it feels as if it does, and this can have a positive knock-on impact on your appetite. While I haven't collated diet data from absolutely everyone in the world, I think I can state with some conviction that most of us eat too much. If you don't believe me, check out the obesity and diabetes figures!

Being satisfied with less food is ultimately a healthy state of being, particularly if we are overweight to begin with.

Nutritional Overload

Detox and cleansing are also a super nutritional program for your body. Consuming a diet consisting entirely of produce gives your anatomy a massive boost of vitamins, minerals, phytonutrients, antioxidants, phenols, and other vital nutrients. Collectively, this will play a large role in helping your body build and repair its depleted systems. You should also feel some benefit in terms of energy production and healing.

This is particularly effective with a detox and cleansing program, as the food involved retains its nutrients that are destroyed in the cooking process. I should mention that there is still some debate over the impact on nutrients from cooking, but there is broad agreement that it has a significant impact.[19]

Additionally, this process enables maximum detoxification of your body to take place. While your anatomy is designed so that it carries this out independently, it also needs some nutritional input. Studies have indicated that the average American has 147 industrial chemicals in their bloodstream,[20] and needless to say, this can mostly be attributed to our toxic diet (although there are other sources, such as medication and commercial toiletries, as well).

Other Physical Benefits

There are several other minor physical benefits of detoxing and cleansing which, when combined, add up to a pretty significant part of the equation. First, those engaging in a juicing program have noticed that their energy levels and thinking have significantly improved. You really do experience a greater clarity of thought. If you stick with the juicing approach, you can expect your energy levels to shoot through the roof in time.

Secondly, those individuals carrying excess weight can certainly expect to lose at least some of it on a juicing program. Some of this will be water weight, but fat will also dissipate as well. Another benefit of detoxing and cleansing is that some of the undesirable physical symptoms that you have experienced previously will diminish, or even disappear. Issues such as headaches, skin rashes, general aches and pains, bloating and trapped gas will all markedly improve as a direct result of this nutritional approach.

Rehydrate Your Body

This one seems rather obvious, but detoxing and cleansing also play a major role in rehydrating the body. This is particularly valuable, as we live in a culture in which there is a level of dehydration that can only be described as chronic. Indeed, a report in 2013 suggested that 75 percent of Americans are chronically dehydrated.[21] Very few people, proportionately, keep themselves properly hydrated, and this has a hugely negative impact on our bodies.

Engaging in a juicing program will ensure that you rehydrate your anatomy, which will bring natural health benefits, as well as an overall feeling of well-being.

Heal Cells

Rehydration will also help cells function more efficiently. This is particularly important, as there are 37 trillion cells in the human body,[22] and each one is effectively a living, breathing entity. It is our cellular health that ultimately defines and determines our external health, so caring for our cells should be a top priority.

An appropriately formulated raw juice cleanse will enable cells to function at an optimal level. This will help create an efficient internal messaging and manufacturing process, which is at the heart of what your body's cells do. As your cellular processes heal, mito-chondria will create energy, free from the usual hassles of fighting off a multitude of free radicals and anatomical inflammation.[23] This will have a huge positive impact on DNA functioning, which will benefit your overall health.

Food Factors

Finally, there are two positive food factors in opting for a detox and cleanse program. First, this process enables you to completely eliminate harmful foods. Dairy, wheat, grains, gluten, additives, herbicides, pesticides, caffeine, alcohol, and other aspects of the diet that can cause problems are completely eradicated. Not only will this improve the level of inflammation in your body, but it will also help you to determine what foods cause you difficulties and discomfort.

For the period of time that you engage in juice cleansing, it will also be easier for you to make food decisions. This can be a weight off your mind in the hectic lives that most of you lead today. Detox-ing keeps you focused on consuming fresh, whole produce every few hours, reducing the anxiety associated with constantly planning out what to eat. You will feel fully satiated in terms of appetite, and it will also demonstrate that it is not necessary to be a slave to harmful food and its ingredients.

The Next Generation

Another reason for doing the detox and cleanse is that it is a chance to educate your children and pass on good habits to the next generation. Remember that much of the food we consume is toxic. Would you like me to list some of the toxic aspects once more? Well, how about herbicides, pesticides, fungicides, wheat, sugar, artificial sweeteners, additives, colorings, saturated fats, trans fats . . . once again, I think you get the general idea!

There is a reason that so many people in our society are unwell, obese, and even increasingly suffer from diabetes. We are stuffing our bodies full of crap! It is that simple! This is our primary health problem in the Western world, and it has so many knock-on effects that are undesirable. By detoxing and cleansing you are flushing all of this garbage out of your system.

Yes, your body will react. It might even react quite strongly. But after seven days you will be in a much better position from a health perspective. You will have a solid foundation to build a new you. The week will absolutely be worth it.

What's a Detox?

Now I know what you're thinking. You're worried about being hungry all the time. I hear you! Well, I've got some good news for you on that score. The nutrient-dense foods you will be consuming during the detox and cleanse process actually help prevent hunger. You will feel full because the quality of food you're getting will simply be far superior to your previous diet. We should definitely favor quality over quantity, right?

Once you create alkalinity within your body and treat it to all the minerals, vitamins, and antioxidants it has been craving, you'll soon feel on top of the world! There is also a lot to be said for benefiting from the energetic frequency contained within the natural food groups that you will be consuming. Tapping into this will make you feel far better than wolfing down a load of stuff that is bad for you and bad for your body. Trust me!

If you trust the internal processes of your body, the process of cleansing, and the process of detox, then your health will improve rapidly, and you will soon feel so good that you will barely be able to believe it. Fresh food is the best food, and you're about to find out how true that is. Detoxing is all about eradicating everything that is bad for your body and only giving it things that it needs and which will benefit its functioning.

The Challenge

Okay, so I have listed many of the benefits of the detox and cleansing process in this chapter. But there is no way of getting around this: you can also expect some side effects. Not everyone will experience these, as everyone's body is different (as I keep saying), and you have all been through completely different environmental experiences and upbringings. Nonetheless, if you have been mistreating your body to a significant degree, you can reasonably expect it to fight back when you detox.

Experiencing mucus buildup, colds, and flu symptoms are very common when detoxing and cleansing for the first time. Essentially, when the body gets a break from dealing with crap, it will naturally and immediately begin to process and rid itself of any waste products. If this sounds in any way unappealing, bear in mind that exactly the same thing happens when you quit smoking. Surely, no one would suggest that this is unhealthy!

Getting Over the Hump

This excess of mucus comes straight from the digestive tract. All you can do is ride it out and let the body do what it needs to in order to heal itself. This will be a challenge, but it is definitely a challenge that can be overcome.

One method that I have found particularly effective is to make yourself a hot water drink with citric juice and ginger. Boil some water, grate some ginger, add it to the water, and finally include the juice of one lime or lemon. Sip on this drink every couple of hours, and you will soon find that the symptoms will ease significantly.

Hunger Problems

Another issue that is particularly common is the body tricking you into wanting to eat solid food. First, I must point out that this is a complete delusion. When on the juicing program, you are easily taking in enough nutrients in order to fuel the body. There is absolutely no physical, anatomical, or biological need for you to consume any form of solid food while on this program.

The reason that your body will tell you that you need to eat solid food is that it feels a psychological compulsion to chew.[24] This is similar to the withdrawal symptoms smokers get when they quit smoking, with the body telling them that they need to do something with their hands and mouth instead. You have been chewing since you were three years old, and psychologically removing yourself from this process will have some impact. Just tell yourself that it makes absolutely no sense. Because it really doesn't!

Food and Emotion

Indeed, all over the world today, and particularly in the Western world, people are shoveling food down their gullets for emotional reasons rather than any objective or rational motivation. This is not necessary! This is not needed! This is definitely not healthy!

When you are engaging in the detox and cleansing process for the first time, try to set aside some time for calmness. Meditate if possible. Try to relish the universal energy that you are taking in from the nutritious food you are consuming, which is connected to the earth and all of its goodness. Realize that all the impulses we have to continually want things are put there by media, and particularly an advertising matrix. You can rise above these impulses and begin to live a healthier and superior existence. I believe in all of you!

Gas and Bloating

Another potential side effect of juicing over an extended period, particularly when this is your first attempt, is gas and bloating.[25] This is quite simply related to cleaning out your trash-can body, which has been a dumpster for all kinds of crap for far too long. In order to address gas and bloating, it is advisable to drink herbal peppermint tea, which will alleviate the symptoms in most cases.

It's important for me to emphasize that you shouldn't add any sweeteners or sugar to peppermint tea or any other drinks that you consume during the detox process. If you do this, you are effectively cheating yourself and defeating the entire detox and cleanse ethos. Stay strong; do not give in to the false impulses of your body and its internal mechanisms. I'll be discussing those more in a bit.

Muscle Mass Myth

One of the myths that many people believe with regard to any detoxing process is that it can result in reduced muscle mass. I feel that this is particularly important to address, as it is a common concern, and also completely untrue!

The fruit and nutrient-packed smoothies and juices that you will be consuming during this detoxing process are absolutely full of proteins and amino acids. There is absolutely no danger of your losing muscle mass during this program. It is worth mentioning that it is practically impossible to lose muscle mass in seven days, anyway.

As mentioned previously, and as I keep saying(!), the human body is an incredible thing and is designed to maintain itself. Your muscles cannot simply dissipate in a matter of days just because you don't eat meat or something! This is just quackery!

Dealing with Eaters!

However, a more practical issue that you will almost inevitably encounter is . . . eaters! Yes, unfortunately there are a lot of them around!

When you are in the vicinity of someone eating something that you especially enjoy, it is obviously quite natural to begin craving food. There is no easy way around this, other than to lock yourself in a dark room for seven days. Of course, this can be difficult from a practical perspective.

So what I suggest instead is simply to step away or step outside when people are eating around you. Don't put yourself through any difficult situations or experiences; simply remove yourself and stick to the program.

Pooping Problems!

Okay, there is no delicate way to say this: you may encounter some toiletry troubles while engaging in this detox process. Pooping may become an issue!

The reason for this is that when you consume juices and smoothies, you are getting around 25 times the level of fiber to which your body is accustomed. This can result in your losing as much as eight pounds of feces during the process. Other people might have the complete opposite reaction and may find it difficult to go to the toilet during the detox and cleanse.

This is perfectly natural. The solid food that comes into your body on a regular basis makes you go to the toilet regularly, and when you eliminate your usual intake of solid food, the digestive system can take a while to adapt.

It is also important to mention that the way we go to the toilet generally should not be considered normal! Think about it. You are constantly eating and yet still completely full of feces. You are going to the toilet several times a day, yet you feel hungry, sick, overweight, have no energy, and are often in an emotional state.

This is because you are filling your body with garbage and are effectively constipated even after you've been to the toilet! Detoxing and cleansing is clearing your body of all this rubbish and resetting your entire digestive tract at the same time that you are repairing your entire cellular system. When you put it like that, isn't it reasonable to expect some period of turbulence?

Enema Value

If you are struggling to go to the toilet during the detoxing program, I always recommend using an enema in order to dislodge excreta. Water is, after all, a solvent, and it will help you get your digestive system squeaky clean.

While we're on the subject, it is also worth mentioning that period pain often emanates from our organs being overloaded with crap.[26] So menstruation can become considerably more bearable if you detox your body. Doesn't that sound like a benefit worth working for?

Cellular Tricks

Now, I realize that some side effects and experiences that you can expect to encounter while engaging in the detox and cleanse process might sound slightly intimidating. So I want to explain and reiterate to you why these things occur and why you should push through some of these negative aspects of the process.

When you engage in a detox and cleanse, you are effectively recalibrating 37 trillion cells. Needless to say, you can expect some internal reaction to this! I'm sure you've heard the expression that every reaction has an equal and opposite reaction. Well, when you change your body to such a fundamental degree, it is only reasonable to expect some sort of reaction from your anatomy.

In your body right now are microbes and bacteria. These are living, breathing organisms that are programmed to fight for survival. They will not be happy as the new alkaline environment within your body destroys them![27] Microbes and bacteria don't like alkalinity. They don't like hydration. They don't like mineralization. They're not getting their drugs and food anymore! So they fight back. They trick your mind and body into feeling that you are dying by depriving yourself of all the things that are ruining your health in the first place. When you feel bad during a detox and cleanse, you are literally feeling what your colon is currently going through. It can be tough.

But it doesn't last forever! I assure you of this. Many people experience a hump on the third day of the cleansing program in particular, but this will soon pass. Detoxing and cleansing helps prevent disease, or even reverse disease, and it keeps you young, healthy, and vital. It is one of the best things that you can ever do for your health, and this is why I absolutely recommend it to all of my clients. It should be the foundation for rebooting your body.

Body Benefits and Oxygenation

Now I want to go into some other benefits of the cleansing process. As the detox occurs, all the organs in your body will open up, as they now have space to breathe, having been freed of the crap that was constricting them. By creating an oxygenated environment, you are really benefiting the functioning of your organs.

Oxygen is also required in order to activate the skin, providing a second elimination channel for any unwanted and unrequired substances. So it is important to get outside three to four times per day and get some sun, as this will really get your whole system moving and also contribute positively to your physical appearance.

Peristaltic Progress

By engaging in this detox and cleanse you are stimulating peristaltic action. This may need a little explanation, as peristalsis is probably something that you haven't encountered before.

The muscles that exist within your esophagus, stomach, small intestine, and colon need to contract and relax in order to digest your food. This process is referred to as peristalsis and is utilized in order to push food through your digestive tract. Any food that you do consume stimulates nerves within this part of the body, and this in turn triggers peristaltic action in these muscles. The type and amount of food that you eat, along with the frequency of each consumption, have an influence on the peristaltic process.[28]

High-fiber foods are among those that stimulate peristalsis,[29] by adding bulk to your daily diet. This penetrates intestinal walls and activates peristaltic activity within the digestive system. Obviously, while you are engaging in the detox and cleanse, the amount of fiber you are consuming is greatly increased over your normal diet. So you can expect a good degree of peristaltic action to occur during this seven-day period.

Why Detox Is Effective

The importance of the gut and of the level of activity that occurs within this system help explain why bloating, gas, and inflammation all stem from the colon. This is why detox is so effective, as it helps to reverse some damaging activity that we tend to engage in on a daily basis.

Detox and cleansing enhance the circulatory system and cleans out the digestive tract.[30] This is really important, as most people's adrenals are completely shot. We have saturated our body with toxins, and now they need water, oxygen, nutrients, sunshine, and sleep; otherwise, the body will simply stop working.

In short, we need to go back to basics, and the detox plan is the first important step in this process.

Busy Gut

We sometimes take for granted the amount of activity that takes place within our bodies, and particularly in our gut and digestive tract. On reflection, this is completely irrational! This is an absolutely critical system of the body, which is simply required in order to survive. Without the energy that we derive from food products, we simply won't be able to function, so it is obvious that the system that regulates this process will need to be pretty active and an important component of the overall anatomy.

Yet many people do not realize that the gut is tight and compact, while the temperature in there is rather hot and humid, not dissimilar to a sauna. In this sort of environment, it is very easy for foodstuffs that you consume to both coagulate and ferment.

It will take your body a little time to get over this, so be patient and allow the natural process of cleansing to unfold.

Hitting the Wall

As I mentioned previously, many people engaging in the detox and cleanse program for the first time experience difficulties on the third day. So if you hit the wall during day three, first, remember that this is perfectly normal. This is really the timeframe that you can expect the microbes and bacteria in your body to begin to fight back against the process of detoxification. After 48 hours, it has sunk into their evil brains that they are being starved to death! They can make you suffer!

What I would recommend at this point is to continually keep yourself hydrated. This is, of course, extremely important anyway, but sometimes the body will cause you problems as it simply requires plain and simple water in order to hydrate. Particularly focus on this process from day three, and you'll find that getting over the hump gets a lot easier.

Consumption Guide

I also want to provide a little guidance regarding how you should consume the juices and smoothies contained within this detox and cleansing program. First, you should aim to consume them within 30 minutes. This should be possible, but at the same time you should bear in mind that you are consuming nutrition-packed food, the likes of which your body may not have encountered for quite some time (if ever).

This means that it can be a little difficult for some people to get the drinks down. But what I would say to you is don't make the process difficult on yourself. You should definitely consume one or two smoothies every day, but if this is proving a struggle, then you shouldn't force them down.

What I would recommend, though, is particularly prioritizing the one that you consume in the morning, as this will elevate your liver function and get the digestive tract working well throughout the day.

Contrast Hydrotherapy

Another valuable technique that certainly merits serious consideration during the detoxing process is contrast hydrotherapy. You may have heard the word *hydrotherapy* used before, but many people do not know too much about it, let alone *contrast hydrotherapy*. In my opinion, this is a hugely effective technique that can be utilized to boost the natural benefits of detox and cleanse further still. But it does require a bit of willpower from you.

Contrast hydrotherapy involves hitting your body with a perpetual combination of cold and hot water. You should first stand under the shower and change the water temperature so that it is piping hot. Allow the water to flow all over your body for 60 seconds, timing this with a mobile device or clock.

Then comes the tricky part! You next turn the shower to cold and allow the cold water to flow over your body for 30 seconds. Lift your arms up so that it goes under your armpits, and try to ensure that your entire body benefits from this bracing experience.

Once you have been through this for 30 seconds, you then switch back to 60 seconds of hot water. The aim is to go through the hot and cold contrast on 10 separate occasions, although this may be somewhat challenging at first. When you're starting out with contrast hydrotherapy, you should instead go through the hot and cold functions for as long as you possibly can.

I guess you're going to want to know the benefits of this before doing it, though! Well, applying warm water to the body results in your blood vessels dilating, which in turn increases blood flow to any affected areas. When cold water is applied, your blood vessels contract. This means that when warm and cold water are used in an alternating fashion, it effectively acts as a pump for your body, tuning your blood vessels and making them more adaptable to physical and emotional stress.[31]

Cold water also activates your sympathetic nervous system,[32] responsible for your body's fight-or-flight response. Stimulating this system will help your body respond flexibly to such stimuli in the future. So when you encounter a fight-or-flight situation from then on, your body won't act as dramatically as it did in the past.

Changing water temperatures also positively impacts the body's energy levels and, overall, can have a significant influence on several aspects of your life and health.

Conclusion

So I hope that I have begun to convince you to engage in a process of detox and cleansing. This will have a beneficial impact on your body and will also make you feel better. I have included some smoothie and juice recipes in the cookbook in order to get you started. I hope this provides you with both motivation and inspiration, although there is nothing stopping you from coming up with your own juice and smoothie ideas as well. Let's do this!

Challenger Story

Tiffany has been one of our success stories with a relatively common tale, but also a unique twist. While Tiffany had experienced problems with her weight, she had also previously had gastric band surgery. So her physical state was significantly different from that of most women.

This meant that while she had put on a bit of weight, she had to be careful of what she did with her body. She perhaps didn't have the freedom that some other women we work with enjoy. But the important thing is that she made the plunge to join this six-week program, which has helped transform her mindset and entire life.

We had to create goals for Tiffany so that she wasn't entirely focused on losing weight. We wanted to focus on personal strength and growth for what were somewhat unusual circumstances.

Many people reading this may not know that gastric band surgery can have an impact on the absorption of iron. This iron deficiency had an impact on Tiffany, and she suffered from bouts of tiredness and lack of energy on a regular basis. So we had a clear incentive to get her life back on track.

Thankfully, we made significant process. The improvement in Tiffany's diet, combined with a personalized training program, improved her health and state of being. For the first time in many years, the mental fog that had been a big part of her life disappeared. Cutting out sugars and carbs, following the dietary program, and exercising as advised . . . and suddenly Tiffany was feeling 100 percent better.

Indeed, she rated her improvement on the six-week program as 10 out of 10! Despite the fact that we never set her specific weight loss goals, she managed to shed 16.4 pounds and 14.6 inches. So although Tiffany's case was a challenging one, the results were better than we'd even hoped.

Tiffany outlined the support she had received during the program as being key to her success. She also mentioned that she had a huge feeling of accomplishment from achieving this physical transformation on her own terms, purely for her own well-being. Her life has been set on a new path, and she has truly learned that her health is nonnegotiable.

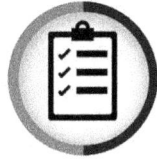

CONCLUSION

So that's a rundown on the best way to take back control of your body and your life. This is something that many of us have needed to do at some stage of our lives. Admitting this to yourself is a critical first step toward turning your life around. Remember the old joke about the psychiatrist and the lightbulb? It only takes one psychiatrist to change a lightbulb, but the lightbulb has to want to change.

Winning the Battle

You want to change, you've made a commitment to changing, and that is half the battle. Many people will live in denial about the deleterious impact that their lifestyles are having on their bodies. Unfortunately, this will have the most serious consequences imaginable. Thankfully, you've made the first step in what will be an empowering journey.

However, don't pat yourselves on the back too firmly! That in itself achieves nothing! You really have to follow through on that initial realization if you're going to whip yourself back into shape. And as I've recounted to you at times during this book, this involves some pain. There is no gain without pain.

But the good news is that the amount of pain you will have to go through is honestly trivial compared to the gain for yourself, your body, and your life. A bit of pain and lots of gain—that's a pretty good deal, right?

Rapid Adaptation

You will find that your body swiftly adapts to what you're doing and that it soon becomes second nature. While there will be a little initial adjustment to some of what you need to do to get yourself back into ship-shape condition, this will pass surprisingly quickly. This is the brilliant thing about the human body. It is adaptable. It is durable. It mends itself. It's definitely the best thing that you will ever have in your life, so you owe it to yourself to take care of it and make sure that it's firing on all cylinders.

This is going to be such a wonderful journey for you. You're going to feel a new vitality driven by the new levels of health and fitness you will experience. I'm super excited about turning more people on to crafting new lives and happiness for themselves.

Toxic Environment

Achieving this has been made so much more difficult by the toxic environment that I have talked about in this book. We live in a climate that systemically makes people end up out of shape, sick, and even dying at a young age. This may be unpalatable, but we shouldn't duck the reality that our lifestyles are literally killing us. You could very well be on the road to that reality right now.

This is why detox and cleansing are so important, as by the time that we've decided to do something about our health, we really need to reverse the damage that we've already done to our bodies. I speak as someone who has had to go through this myself, as well as someone who has, by now, helped countless people through the same process.

Your health is nonnegotiable, and that means you have to recalibrate your entire existence.

Upside-Down, Inside-Out

And there is something deeply ironic about this entire process. At first, what you are doing may seem abnormal and will almost certainly be somewhat foreign. However, in reality, it is actually perfectly logical and indeed normal. Conversely, what contemporary society and culture have taught us to do with our bodies is actually completely unhealthy. Our "sophisticated" way of living has turned what is normal completely on its head, and now the abnormal has instead been normalized.

If we were living in a healthy society now, we wouldn't have to go through this program in the first place. I wouldn't say that absolutely no one would have had to have done this in the past, and I'm sure even then many people would have benefited from it. But you really don't need to go back that many years in order to experience a time in which many people were fundamentally healthier.

Those defending our lifestyles today will tend to point to the life expectancy of the human race increasing as evidence that the way we live is not so bad. But this is hugely misleading for several reasons.

Societal Trends

We simply cannot discount the rapidly evolving technology and state of society that have occurred over the previous decades when considering this issue. Many diseases have been completely eradicated, or at the very least marginalized in terms of being life-threatening. This is largely due to the development of medicine, while massively improved sanitation conditions have also had a vast influence. Even the refrigeration of food has played a prominent role.

Additionally, life expectancy is hugely influenced by the level of infant mortality, and this rate has rapidly declined over the last 100 years. At one time it was almost normal for a young child or baby to pass away; whereas we now expect our infants to make it through their early lives unscathed. Indeed, as noted by Slate: "Because the bulk of human mortality occurs at young and old ages, life expectancy is heavily influenced by child death rates . . . much of that increase is thanks to falling death rates among women and young children, especially from infectious diseases."[1]

It should also be noted that life expectancy certainly isn't increasing everywhere, and there has been a broad trend of this figure reaching a plateau, or even declining. A recent CDC report indicated that life expectancy in the United States has declined for two consecutive years. This is the first time this has occurred since the 1960s, and this was due to an influenza outbreak.[2] Statistics Canada also reported recently that life expectancy has basically plateaued for Canadians.[3]

Inequality and Lifestyle

While *The Washington Post* blamed these figures on a "drug crisis,"[4] a more realistic citation of inequality was made by Vox.[5] This latter suggestion was also backed up by data from Public Health England and the Office for National Statistics in Britain, which concluded that there were "alarming disparities in longevity" based on the geographical region in which people are resident.[6]

Obviously, inequality doesn't literally cause premature death. It is just more likely that relatively impoverished people will not look after themselves as well or exercise their bodies as regularly, and they will eat worse food, more often—comfort eating with increased regularity. That adds up to a noxious cocktail that is killing people. This cannot be denied. The figures are quite clear.

Aside from life expectancy, another key point is: life cannot be judged by merely being alive! Surely there is more to life than simply surviving! We should be thriving in this modern world in which many of the vicious diseases that killed people in the past have been rendered obsolete.

Yet for many people, their organs are simply keeping them alive. They tick from day to day, but their bodies are a mess, they feel terrible, and they look bad. Is this what life should look like in the most technologically advanced society in human history? Should we really be experiencing unprecedented levels of obesity and diabetes in such a culture?

I will say once again that if this were a healthy society, we wouldn't have to reboot our bodies. So the ethos of what I'm outlining in this book is about becoming normal and healthy again. It's as simple as that.

Targeting Inflammation

It should be remembered that inflammation in the body is fundamental to a great deal of the problems and poor health that people experience. If you haven't been looking after yourself satisfactorily, you will be inflamed internally. Beginning to turn the tide on inflammation will make such a difference to your health, and ultimately your life.

Most health problems can usually be traced back to this condition. Indeed, inflammation is the body's method of indicating that it has a problem in the first place! Reducing, and then eliminating, inflammation will be a massive kick-start to your whole anatomy. This is why it should always be a central focus of your approach to health and well-being.

Gut Gripes

Equally, many people in Western society have poor gut health. We undoubtedly bombard our guts with crap on an almost daily basis. Yet this criminally neglected aspect of our bodies is critical to our well-being. Microbial research is demonstrating that the gut may be even more important than we understood previously. So recalibrating your gut, and ensuring that it is healthy going forward, will really reap rewards.

Great Results

There are many problems in this world, and our diets and general health are certainly among the most worrisome. But what I can tell you is that you're going to get great results from following this program. Your inflamed body will calm down, your gut health will drastically improve, and eventually your entire outlook and existence will be greatly enhanced.

Being involved in this line of work has undoubtedly been the best thing that has ever happened to me. It is so life-affirming and inspiring to encounter people turning around their entire existences from positions where they were really depressed and unwell.

Turning the Tide

Something else I'd like to emphasize as well is that not only will you get a physical boost from engaging in this new healthy lifestyle, but your self-esteem will be greatly enhanced as well. You will become a new person: Yourself 2.0!

You will remain motivated because your life will be better. What once seemed unnatural will now seem natural, and you will wonder how and why you ever engaged in the toxic lifestyle you followed previously. After all, what could be more natural than looking good and feeling great? That's what I want for everyone who reads this book, and it's within your reach to achieve it.

I'd like to remind you that science is always leading us down new paths of exploration, and there is always something new to learn. I make it my business to stay up to date on the latest science and the studies that continue to lead us down a new path. I do not teach the same lessons as I did 10 years ago, and I know I will certainly adjust my opinions down the road as science unfolds new discoveries about the body.

Even as I write this final chapter, I'm learning about how the microbiome and the bacteria in our bodies are extremely different from one body to another. It is largely the microbiome and the varied combination of the bacteria that ultimately determine whether one person can eat broccoli while another cannot, or why some cancer treatment medications work for some versus being ineffective to others.

It's fascinating to learn that your own microbiome changes constantly as your body lives in the world and is exposed to different bacteria entering and dying within the body. It's been suggested that the human body is simply a shell that houses the trillions of bacteria and that it's the bacteria that governs our every move. It's a futuristic concept that you might watch in a sci-fi movie, but this concept makes perfect sense to me. It's a fascinating topic, and I encourage you to dive deeper into the science if you feel the motivation.

On that note, I want to also remind you that your body's genetic and bacterial makeup is so very different from anyone else's. So it absolutely will require you to roll up your sleeves to understand what works and what doesn't work for your body when it comes to fitness and nutrition. I can offer you a variety of tests to measure gut health, food sensitivities, metals, hormone regulation, stress, and of course your DNA, but simple trial-and-error experimentation can often give you all the information you need. It's time to put on your lab coat and geek out on yourself.

The choice is yours.

NOTES

CHAPTER TWO

1. Jason Fung, MD, "Fasting Lowers Cholesterol – Fasting 16," (2017), https://idmprogram.com/fasting-lowers-cholesterol-fasting-16.

2. "Could you lower your blood pressure through fasting?" (2018), https://www.health24.com/Medical/Hypertension/Lifestyle-changes/Hypertension-and-fasting-20120721.

3. Salah M. Aly, PhD, "Role of Intermittent Fasting on Improving Health and Reducing Diseases," (2014), https://www.ncbi.nlm.nih.gov/pmc/articles/PMC4257368.

4. (2017), https://www.buchinger-wilhelmi.com/en.

5. Björn A. Menge, L. Grüber, S. M. Jørgensen, C. F. Deacon, W. E. Schmidt, J. D. Veldhuis, J. J. Holst, and J. J. Meier, "Loss of inverse relationship between pulsatile insulin and glucagon secretion in patients with type 2 diabetes," (2011), https://www.ncbi.nlm.nih.gov/pubmed/21677283.

6. Suzanne Wu, "Fasting triggers stem cell regeneration of damaged, old immune system," (2014), https://news.usc.edu/63669.

7. "The Effects of Fasting Ketosis," (2017), https://www.allaboutfasting.com/effects-of-fasting-ketosis.html.

8. Kristina Fiore, "Skipping Meals May Shed Lbs., Boost Brain," (2013), https://www.medpagetoday.com/meetingcoverage/obesityweek/42966.

9. Jason Fung, MD, "Fasting Physiology – Part II," (2016), https://idmprogram.com/fasting-physiology-part-ii.

10. Thai Nguyen, "10 Proven Ways to Grow Your Brain: Neurogenesis and Neuroplasticity," (2017), http://theutopianlife.com/2016/05/31/3094.

11. Valter Longo, PhD, "Valter Longo - Fasting Mimicking Diet & Your Immune System," (2018), https://www.youtube.com/watch?v=vdjG-grh5zSk.

12. Sarah Knapton, "Fasting for three days can regenerate entire immune system, study finds," (2014), https://www.telegraph.co.uk/science/2016/03/12/fasting-for-three-days-can-regenerate-entire-immune-system-study.

13. Emily Gersema, "Fasting-like diet turns the immune system against cancer," (2016), https://news.usc.edu/103972.

14. Changhan Lee, L. Raffaghello, S. Brandhorst, F. M. Safdie, G. Bianchi,

A. Martin-Montalvo, V. Pistoia, M. Wei, S. Hwang, A. Merlino, L. Emionite, R. de Cabo, and V. D. Longo, "Fasting cycles retard growth of tumors and sensitize a range of cancer cell types to chemotherapy," (2012), https://www.ncbi.nlm.nih.gov/pubmed/22323820.

15. "Fasting can trigger stem cell, immune regeneration," (2017), https://spinalresearch.com.au/fasting-can-trigger-stem-cell-immune-regeneration.

16. "Intermittent Fasting for Leaky Gut, Rapid Healing, and Weight Loss," (2017), https://www.glutenfreesociety.org/intermittent-fasting-for-leaky-gut-rapid-healing-and-weight-loss.

17. Rich Haridy, "Harvard study uncovers why fasting can lead to a longer and healthier life," (2017), https://newatlas.com/52058.

18. Jason Fung, MD, "How fasting affects your physiology and hormones," (2016), https://www.dietdoctor.com/fasting-affects-physiology-hormones.

19. Fran Lowry, "Alternate-Day Fasting Poses No Threat to Bone Health," (2016), https://www.medscape.com/viewarticle/870351.

CHAPTER THREE

1. T. R. Reid, "How We Spend $3,400,000,000,000," (2017), https://www.theatlantic.com/health/archive/2017/06/how-we-spend-3400000000000/530355.

2. "Heart Disease Facts," (2018), https://www.cdc.gov/heartdisease/facts.htm.

3. Zosia Chustecka, "Cancer Strikes 1 in 2 Men and 1 in 3 Women," (2007), https://www.medscape.com/viewarticle/551998.

4. "Breast Cancer Facts," (2017), https://www.nationalbreastcancer.org/breast-cancer-facts.

5. Super Size Me, (produced by The Con, 2004).

6. Raymond N. Dubois, "The Jeremiah Metzger Lecture: Inflammation, Immune Modulators, and Chronic Disease," (2015), https://www.ncbi.nlm.nih.gov/pubmed/26330682.

7. Kamila Sitwell, "Typical sugar consumption now vs 100 years ago," (2016), www.divineeatingout.com/food-1/sugar-consumption-now-vs-100-years-ago.

8. "Trans fat is double trouble for your heart health," (2017), https://newsnetwork.mayoclinic.org/discussion/transfat-is-double-trouble-for-your-heart-health.

9. Adda Bjarnadottir, "Why Refined Carbs Are Bad for You," (2017), https://www.healthline.com/nutrition/why-refined-carbs-are-bad.

10. B. Boyers, "GMOs and Pesticides—What Concerns Scientists," (2011), calmfulliving.org/project/gmos-and-pesticides-what-concerns-scientists.

11. "Animal Feed," (2018), www.sustainabletable.org/260/animal-feed.

12. McLibel, (produced by Spanner Films, 2005).

13. Rachel Link, RD, "Cruciferous Vegetables: Cancer Killer or Thyroid Killer?" (2017), https://draxe.com/cruciferous-vegetables-cancer-thyroid.

14. N. Fujioka, V. Fritz, P. Upadhyaya, F. Kassie, and S. S. Hecht, "Research on cruciferous vegetables, indole-3-carbinol, and cancer prevention: A tribute to Lee W. Wattenberg," (2016), https://www.ncbi.nlm.nih.gov/pubmed/26840393.

15. J. Luis Espinoza, L. Q. Trung, P. T. Inaoka, K. Yamada, D. T. An, S. Mizuno, S. Nakao, and A. Takami, "The Repeated Administration of Resveratrol Has Measurable Effects on Circulating T-Cell Subsets in Humans," (2017), https://www.hindawi.com/journals/omcl/2017/6781872.

16. Mark Sisson, "Fall Foods: Why Seasonal Eating Primes the Body for Fat Burning," (2012), https://www.marksdailyapple.com/fall-foods-why-seasonal-eating-primes-the-body-for-fat-burning.

17. Joseph R. Hibbelna and Rachel V. Gow, "Omega-3 fatty acid and nutrient deficits in adverse neurodevelopment and childhood behaviors," (2014), https://www.ncbi.nlm.nih.gov/pubmed/24975625.

18. A. P. Simopolous, "Omega-3 fatty acids in inflammation and autoimmune diseases," (2002), https://www.ncbi.nlm.nih.gov/pubmed/12480795.

CHAPTER FOUR

1. Alison Abbott, "Scientists bust myth that our bodies have more bacteria than human cells," (2016), https://www.nature.com/news/1.19136.

2. Christopher Bergland, "Gut Microbiota May Influence Mood and Behavior, Study Finds," (2017), https://www.psychologytoday.com/us/blog/the-athletes-way/201706/gut-microbiota-may-influence-mood-and-behavior-study-finds.

3. Megan Clapp, N. Aurora, L. Herrera, M. Bhatia, E. Wilen, and S. Wakefield, "Gut microbiota's effect on mental health: The gut-brain axis," (2017), https://www.ncbi.nlm.nih.gov/pmc/articles/PMC5641835.

4. Jamie Morea, "The Link between Gut Health and Stress," (2017), https://medium.com/thrive-global/682aafa355c7.

5. "Can Genetics Explain an Unhealthy Gut?" (2016), https://bodyecology.com/articles/can-genetics-explain-an-unhealthy-gut.

6. "Facts about Antibiotic Resistance," (2016), https://www.cdc.gov/antibiotic-use/community/about/fast-facts.html.

7. "The 7 Most Common Causes of Candida," (2018), https://www.thecandidadiet.com/causes-of-candida.

8. "Addiction to Cheese Is Real Thanks to Casomorphins," (2016), https://yumuniverse.com.

9. J Dolm, "A 12-Step Guide to Kicking that Cheese Addiction," (2016), www.onegreenplanet.org/vegan-food.

10. Amy Myers, MD, "The Problem with Grains and Legumes," (2014), https://www.amymyersmd.com.

11. John Douillard, "Understanding Gluten and How to Digest It," (2014), https://lifespa.com/understanding-gluten-digest.

12. "11 Ways Gluten and Wheat Can Damage Your Health," (2018), https://paleoleap.com/11-ways-gluten-and-wheat-can-damage-your-health.

13. Chris Kresser, "The Thyroid-Gut Connection," (2010), https://chriskesser.com/the-thyroid-gut-connection.

14. "Facts and Statistics," (2017), https://www.foodallergy.org/life-with-food-allergies/food-allergy-101/facts-and-statistics.

15. Susan Blum, MD, "Leaky Gut and Food Sensitivities," (2017), https://blumhealthmd.com/2017/07/25/leaky-gut-and-food-sensitivities.

16. "Rheumatoid Arthritis Facts and Statistics," (2017), https://www.rheumatoidarthritis.org/ra/facts-and-statistics.

17. "The 4 Most Common Deficiencies & How to Love Your Liver," (2017), https://thewholejourney.com/liver-health-glutathione-and-vitamin-mineral-deficiencies-lauren-noel-n-d.

18. "The Gut-Skin Connection," (2017), https://tailorskin.co/blogs/news/all-natural.

19. Tom Bayne, "Fiber and Probiotics: Why This Little-Known Combination Is Key for Good Digestive Health," (2011), https://pbhealthcenter.com/2011/09/fiber-and-probiotics-why-this-little-known-combination-is-key-for-good-digestive-health.

20. RadhaKrishna Rao and Geetha Samak, "Role of Glutamine in Protection of Intestinal Epithelial Tight Junctions," (2015), https://

www.ncbi.nlm.nih.gov/pmc/articles/PMC4369670.

21. Laurell Matthews, ND, "N-acetylglucosamine for Rebuilding the Gut," (2015), https://drlaurell.com/2015/04/20/n-acetylglucosamine-for-rebuilding-the-gut.

22. Daiki Kubomura, T. Ueno, M. Yamada, A. Tomonaga, and I. Nagaoka, "Effect of N-acetylglucosamine administration on cartilage metabolism and safety in healthy subjects without symptoms of arthritis: A case report," (2017), https://www.ncbi.nlm.nih.gov/pubmed/28413518.

23. "Quercetin: Overview," (2015), pennstatehershey.adam.com/content. aspx?productId=107&pic=33&gid=000322.

24. "Hydrochloric Acid (HCl) and Enzymes for Digestion," (2017), https://functionalhealthminute.com/2017/02/hydrochloric-acid-hcl-and-enzymes-for-digestion.

CHAPTER FIVE

1. Eun Joo Kim, B. Pellman, and J. Kim, "Stress effects on the hippocampus: a critical review," (2015), https://www.ncbi.nlm.nih.gov/pmc/articles/PMC4561403.

2. Jane Collingwood, "The Power of Music to Reduce Stress," (2018), https://psychcentral.com/lib/the-power-of-music-to-reduce-stress.

3. X. Han, J. Gibson, D. L. Eggett, and T. L. Parker, "Bergamot (Citrus bergamia) Essential Oil Inhalation Improves Positive Feelings in the Waiting Room of a Mental Health Treatment Center: A Pilot Study," (2017), https://www.ncbi.nlm.nih.gov/pubmed/28337799.

4. J. D. Amsterdam, J. Shults, I. Soeller, J. J. Mao, K. Rockwell, and A. B. Newberg, "Chamomile (Matricaria recutita) may provide antidepressant activity in anxious, depressed humans: an exploratory study," (2012), https://www.ncbi.nlm.nih.gov/pubmed/22894890.

5. J. Hellhammer, T. Hero, N. Franz, C. Contreras, and M. Schubert, "Omega-3 fatty acids administered in phosphatidylserine improved certain aspects of high chronic stress in men," (2012), https://www.ncbi.nlm.nih.gov/pubmed/22575036.

6. P. Monteleone, M. Maj, L. Beinat, M. Natale, and D. Kemali, "Blunting by chronic phosphatidylserine administration of the stress-induced activation of the hypothalamo-pituitary-adrenal axis in healthy men," (1992), https://www.ncbi.nlm.nih.gov/pubmed/1325348.

7. Carly Fraser, "New Study: Magnesium Found to Treat Depression Better than Antidepressant Drugs," (2017), https://livelovefruit.com/magnesium-treats-depression-better-than-antidepressant-drugs.

8. "Stress and Your Kidneys," (2017), https://www.kidney.org/atoz/content/Stress_and_your_Kidneys.

9. Fawne Hansen, "How Does Stress Affect Your Immune System?" (2017), https://adrenalfatiguesolution.com/stress-immune-system.

10. Michael Lam, MD, MPH, J. Lam, and C. Lam, MD, "Chronic Inflammation and Adrenal Fatigue Part 1," (2016), https://www.drlam.com/chronic-inflammation-and-adrenal-fatigue-part-1.

11. Lindsay Holmes, "5 Ways Stress Wrecks Your Sleep (and What to Do about It)," (2014), https://www.huffingtonpost.com/2014/09/17/stress-and-sleep_n_5824506.html.

12. Ibid.

13. Elizabeth Scott, "How Stress Can Cause a Low Libido," (2017), https://www.verywellmind.com/how-stress-can-lead-to-low-libido-3145029.

14. "Stress in America: The State of Our Nation," (2017), https://www.apa.org/news/press/releases/stress/2017/state-nation.pdf.

15. Victoria Larned, "Obesity among all US adults reaches all-time high," (2013), https://www.cnn.com/2017/10/13/health/adult-obesity-increase-study/index.html.

16. "Measured body mass index, Canadian Community Health Survey – Nutrition, 2015," (2015), https://www150.statcan.gc.ca/n1/en/daily-quotidien/170801/dq170801a-eng.pdf?st=8Ec1p1Ji.

17. Sarah L. Teegarden and T. Bale, "Effects of stress on dietary preference and intake are dependent on access and stress sensitivity," (2008), https://www.ncbi.nlm.nih.gov/pmc/articles/PMC2483328.

18. Deane Alban and P. Alban, "12 Effects of Chronic Stress on Your Brain," (2017), https://bebrainfit.com/effects-chronic-stress-brain.

19. Chris Iliades, MD, "How Stress Affects Digestion," (2018), https://www.everydayhealth.com/hs/better-digestion/how-stress-affects-digestion.

20. Marissa Maldonado, "How Stress Affects Mental Health," (2014), https://psychcentral.com/blog/how-stress-affects-mental-health.

21. "Uncovering the link between emotional stress and heart disease," (2017), https://www.health.harvard.edu/heart-disease-overview/uncovering-the-link-between-emotional-stress-and-heart-disease.

22. Ian Sample, "Stressful jobs double risk of depression for young workers," (2007), https://www.theguardian.com/science/2007/aug/02/mentalhealth.workplacestress.

23. Kate Kelland, "Nearly 40 percent of Europeans suffer mental illness,"

(2011), https://www.reuters.com/article/us-europe-mental-illness/nearly-40-percent-of-europeans-suffer-mental-illness-idUS-TRE7832JJ20110904.

24. Pamela Cowan, "Depression will be the second leading cause of disease by 2020: WHO," (2010), www.calgaryherald.com/health/Depression+will+second+leading+cause+disease+2020/3640325/story.html.

25. Douglas Main, "30 Percent of Americans Have Had an Alcohol-Use Disorder," (2015), https://www.newsweek.com/30-percent-americans-have-had-alcohol-use-disorder-339085.

26. "Results from the 2010 National Survey on Drug Use and Health: Summary of National Findings," (2011), https://www.samhsa.gov/data/sites/default/files/NSDUHNationalFindingsResults2010-web/2k10ResultsRev/NSDUHresultsRev2010.pdf.

27. J. E. Mawdsley and D. S. Rampton, "Psychological stress in IBD: new insights into pathogenic and therapeutic implications," (2005), https://ncbi.nlm.nih.gov/pubmed/16162953.

28. Chris Iliades, MD, "How Stress Affects Digestion," (2018), https://www.everydayhealth.com/hs/better-digestion/how-stress-affects-digestion.

29. Jamie Morea, "The Link between Gut Health and Stress," (2017), https://medium.com/thrive-global/the-link-between-gut-health-and-stress-682aafa355c7.

30. "Blood Sugar & Stress," (2018), https://dtc.ucsf.edu/types-of-diabetes/type2/understanding-type-2-diabetes/how-the-body-processes-sugar/blood-sugar-stress.

31. Melanie Greenberg, PhD, "Why We Gain Weight When We're Stressed—And How Not To," (2013), https://www.psychologytoday.com/us/blog/the-mindful-self-express/201308/why-we-gain-weight-when-we-re-stressed-and-how-not.

32. Ann S. Barnes, MD, "The Epidemic of Obesity and Diabetes: Trends and Treatments," (2011), https://www.ncbi.nlm.nih.gov/pmc/articles/PMC3066828.

33. Korin Miller, "Stress Diarrhea and Constipation: Why Stress Messes with Your Poop," (2017), https://www.self.com/story/stress-diarrhea-and-constipation.

34. Saul McLeod, "Stress, Illness and the Immune System," (2010), https://www.simplypsychology.org/stress-immune.html.

35. Harry Mills, PhD, N. Reiss, PhD, and M. Dombeck, PhD, "Mental and Emotional Impact of Stress," (2008), https://www.mentalhelp.net/articles/mental-and-emotional-impact-of-stress.

CHAPTER SIX

1. Mirel Ketchiff, "The Sleep and Exercise Connection that Can Change Your Life and Your Workouts," (2017), https://www.shape.com/fitness/tips/sleep-and-exercise-connection-that-can-change-your-life-and-your-workouts.

2. Erin Brodwin, "Here's Why You Should Never Eat Right before Bed," (2016), https://www.sciencealert.com/here-s-why-you-should-never-eat-right-before-bed.

3. Owen Bond, "How Caffeine Affects the Nervous System," (2017), https://www.livestrong.com/article/409740/how-caffeine-affects-the-nervous -system.

4. Denise Mann, "Alcohol and a Good Night's Sleep Don't Mix," (2013), https://www.webmd.com/sleep-disorders/news/20130118/alcohol-sleep#1.

5. "How Meditation Boosts Melatonin, Serotonin, GABA, DHEA, Endorphins, Growth Hormone & More," (2018), https://ecoinstitute.org/meditation/dhea_gaba_cortisol_hgh_melatonin_serotonin_endorphins.

6. "The 5 Health Benefits of Having an Orgasm," (2011), https://www.self.com/story/the-5-health-benefits-of-havin.

7. "The Physiology of Sleep: Thermoregulation & Sleep," (2017), sleepdisorders.sleepfoundation.org/chapter-1-normal-sleep/the-physiology-of-sleep-thermoregulation-sleep.

8. Alyse Wexler, "Does valerian root treat anxiety treatment and insomnia?" (2017), https://www.medicalnewstoday.com/articles/318088.php.

9. "Herbs & the Nervous System," (2018), https://www.traditionalmedicinals.com/articles/herbs-nervous-system.

10. "Health Benefits of Magnesium," (2017), https://www.ancient-minerals.com/magnesium-benefits/health.

11. Adda Bjarnadottir, "7 Nutrient Deficiencies that Are Incredibly Common," (2015), https://www.healthline.com/nutrition/7-common-nutrient-deficiencies.

12. "Understanding L-theanine: Sleep better at night, feel relaxed and alert during the day," (2017), https://www.thesleepdoctor.com/2017/07/11/understanding-l-theanine-sleep-better-night-feel-relaxed-alert-day.

13. Angela Sanford, "Brain Benefits of L-Theanine," (2016), https://www.lifeextension.com/Magazine/2016/3/Brain-Benefits-of-L-Theanine/Page-01.

14. "Kava Root: Do the Risks Outweigh the Benefits?" (2017), https://

draxe.com/kava-root.

15. "Cortisol and Morning Energy," (2017), https://www.wellnessresources. com/health-topics/adrenals/cortisol.

16. "Sleep-Wake Cycle: Its Physiology and Impact on Health," (2006), https://sleepfoundation.org/sites/default/files/SleepWakeCycle.pdf.

17. K. L. Knuston and E. Van Cauter, "Associations between sleep loss and increased risk of obesity and diabetes," (2008), https://www.ncbi.nlm. nih.gov/pubmed/18591489.

18. John Von Radowitz, "Alzheimer's Linked to Poor Sleep Patterns in New Study," (2017), https://www.independent.co.uk/life-style/ health-and-families/health-news/alzheimers-disease-sleep-study-neu-rology-research-university-wisconsin-madison-barbara-bend-lin-a7826681.html.

19. "What's the difference between a catabolic and anabolic state?" (2016), https://straighthealth.com/whats-the-difference-between-a-catabol-ic-and-anabolic-state.

20. "Melatonin and Sleep," (2018), https://www.sleepfoundation.org/ sleep-topics/melatonin-and-sleep.

21. G. M. Brown, "Light, melatonin and the sleep-wake cycle," (1994), https://www.ncbi.nlm.nih.gov/pmc/articles/PMC1188623.

22. Arjun Walia, "How to Absorb Earth's Free Flowing Electrons through the Soles of Your Feet (Earthing)," (2016), https://www.collective-evo-lution.com/2016/10/12/earthing-how-to-absorb-earths-free-flowing-electrons-through-the-soles-of-your-feet.

23. "The Frequency of Life," (2017), drjoedispenza.net/blog/health/the-frequency-of-life.

CHAPTER SEVEN

1. Patricia Ramos, "10 Simple Ways to Detox Your Liver," (2017), https:// detoxdiy.com/how-to-detox-your-liver.

2. John Lee, "How's Your Liver? 8 Ways to Mend Your Liver after Quitting Alcohol," (2017), https://www.choosehelp.com/topics/ alcoholism/understanding-alcoholic-liver-disease-and-cirrhosis.

3. Kellyann Petrucci, "A 30-Day Detox to Fight Aging & Reduce Inflammation," (2015), https://www.mindbodygreen.com/0-16854/a-30day-detox-to-fight-aging-reduce-inflammation.html.

4. D. Julien, "8 Detox Symptoms That Show Your Cleanse Is Working," (2017), https://omdetox.com/8-detox-symptoms.

5.   Jessica Bruso, "Anti-Inflammation Diet for Osteoarthritis," (2017), https://healthfully.com/88583-antiinflammation-diet-osteoarthritis.html.

6.   Andy Hnilo, "Want Beautiful Skin? Take Care of Your Liver," (2017), https://alituranaturals.com/want-beautiful-skin-take-care-liver.

7.   Charlotte Watson, "The 7-day anti-ageing detox," (2012), https://www.netdoctor.co.uk/healthy-eating/a10903/the-7-day-anti-ageing-detox.

8.   Alexis Chateau, "Heavy Metal Detox: 10 Things You Can Do to Give Your Body a Lift," (2017), https://www.honeycolony.com/article/heavy-metal-detox.

9.   Karen Wojciechowski, "Brain Fog Causes, Symptoms & Solutions," (2018), https://www.linkedin.com/pulse/brain-fog-causes-symptoms-solutions-karen-wojciechowski.

10. A. Duran, "How to Heal from Depression and Anxiety Naturally," (2018), https://www.spiritrawpicalhealing.com/single-post/2018/02/09/How-To-Heal-From-Depression-and-Anxiety-Naturally.

11. Ana Sandoiu, "Lactate may be key for cancer development," (2017), https://www.medicalnewstoday.com/articles/316438.php.

12. Veronique Desaulniers, "Chemotherapy Detox: How to Rebuild Your Health after Chemo," (2017), https://thetruthaboutcancer.com/chemotherapy-detox.

13. Deepak Chopra, "Weekly Health Tip: When Heartburn Becomes a Health Problem," (2017), https://www.huffingtonpost.com/deepak-chopra/heartburn-gerd_b_931382.html.

14. Lindsay Boyers, "Acids That Are Important to the Human Body," (2018), https://healthyeating.sfgate.com/acids-important-human-body-9207.html.

15. John F. Cryan, PhD, "Toward Psychobiotics: The Microbiome as a Key Regulator of Brain and Behavior," (2015), https://nccih.nih.gov/training/videolectures/towards-psychobiotics.

16. Amy Fleming, "Is your gut microbiome the key to health and happiness?" (2017), https://www.theguardian.com/lifeandstyle/2017/nov/06/microbiome-gut-health-digestive-system-genes-happiness.

17. Catherine Guthrie, "How to Heal a Leaky Gut," (2015), https://experiencelife.com/article/how-to-heal-a-leaky-gut.

18. Woodson Merrell, MD, "The Real Reasons Juice Cleanses Can Get Your Health Back on Track," (2014), https://www.huffingtonpost.com/woodson-merrell-md/juice-cleanses_b_4549641.html.

19. Franziska Spritzler, "How Cooking Affects the Nutrient Content of Foods," (2016), https://www.healthline.com/nutrition/

cooking-nutrient-content.

20. Rebecca Ruiz, "Industrial Chemicals Lurking in Your Bloodstream," (2010), https://www.forbes.com/2010/01/21/toxic-chemicals-bpa-lifestyle-health-endocrine-disruptors.html#9c0ce9bbb91c.

21. John Ericson, "75% of Americans May Suffer from Chronic Dehydration, According to Doctors," (2013), https://www.medicaldaily.com/75-americans-may-suffer-chronic-dehydration-according-doctors-247393.

22. Rose Eveleth, "There Are 37.2 Trillion Cells in Your Body," (2013), https://www.smithsonianmag.com/smart-news/there-are-372-trillion-cells-in-your-body-4941473.

23. "Mitochondria," (2014), https://www.nature.com/scitable/topicpage/mitochondria-14053590.

24. Marc David, "The Psychology of Chewing," (2013), psychologyofeating.com/psychobiology-chewing.

25. Amy Lucas, "Side Effects of a 7-Day Detox," (2017), https://www.livestrong.com/article/152166-side-effects-of-a-7-day-detox.

26. Sacha Strebe, "PMS: What It Is, Why We Get It, and How to Treat It," (2017), https://www.mydomaine.com/how-to-treat-pms-symptoms.

27. Keith Bell, "Drink High Alkaline Water to Raise Protective Gut Microbiota," (2016), thegutclub.org/2016/12/22/drink-high-alkaline-water-to-raise-protective-gut-microbiota.

28. Michelle Matte, "Are There Certain Foods That Stimulate Peristaltic Motion?" (2017), https://www.livestrong.com/article/517213-foods-that-stimulate-peristaltic-motion.

29. Sandi Busch, "Foods That Stimulate Peristaltic Motion," (2017), https://healthyeating.sfgate.com/foods-stimulate-peristaltic-motion-11787.html.

30. Jon Barron, "Colon Cleanse: Death Begins in the Colon," (2011), https://jonbarron.org/article/death-begins-colon.

31. Paul Ingraham, "Contrast Hydrotherapy: "Exercising" tissues with quick changes in temperature, to help with pain and injury rehab (especially repetitive strain injuries)," (2015), https://www.painscience.com/articles/contrasting.php.

32. Michael Sieber, "The Benefits of Taking Cold Showers," (2014), https://www.thefunctionalbody.com/the-benefits-of-taking-cold-showers.

CONCLUSION

1. Ben Hanowell, "Life Expectancy Is, Overall, Increasing," (2016), www.slate.com/articles/health_and_science/medical_examiner/2016/12/life_expectancy_is_still_increasing.html.

2. Robin L. Smith, "US Life Expectancy Declines Two Years in a Row," (2018), https://www.huffingtonpost.com/entry/us-life-expectancy-declines-two-years-in-a-row_us_5a5f8582e4b067e1058ff146.

3. S. Boesveld, "As life expectancy growth slows in Canada, are our lifespans hitting the 'wall of death' limit?" (2014), https://nationalpost.com/news/canada/as-life-expectancy-growth-slows-in-canada-are-our-lifespans-hitting-the-wall-of-death-limit.

4. L. Bernstein and C. Ingraham, "Fueled by drug crisis, U.S. life expectancy declines for a second straight year," (2017), https://www.washingtonpost.com/national/health-science/fueled-by-drug-crisis-us-life-expectancy-declines-for-a-second-straight-year/2017/12/20/2e3f-8dea-e596-11e7-ab50-621fe0588340_story.html?noredirect=on&utm_term=.fe4c46fdd18a.

5. J. Belluz, "What the dip in US life expectancy is really about: inequality," (2018), https://www.vox.com/science-and-health/2018/1/9/16860994/life-expectancy-us-income-inequality.

6. L. Pasha-Robinson, "Life expectancy plummets in parts of UK, data reveals," (2018), https://www.independent.co.uk/news/uk/home-news/life-expectancy-uk-plumments-ons-data-hartlepool-torridge-amber-valley-barnsley-a8164171.html.